D1293113

Controlling Medical Professionals

Controlling Medical Professionals

The Comparative Politics of Health Governance

edited by
Giorgio Freddi and
James Warner Björkman

SAGE Modern Politics Series Volume 21
Sponsored by the European Consortium for
Political Research/ECPR

S SAGE Publications
London · Newbury Park · New Delhi

SAGE Publications Ltd
28 Banner Street
London EC1Y 8QE

SAGE Publications Inc
2111 West Hillcrest Drive
Newbury Park, California 91320

SAGE Publications India Pvt Ltd
32, M-Block Market
Greater Kailash - I
New Delhi 110 048

British Library Cataloguing in Publication data

Controlling medical professionals: the comparative
   politics of health governance.–
   (Sage modern politics series; 21)
   1. Health services. Administration. Political
   aspects
   I. Freddi, Giorgio   II. Björkman, James Warner
   362.1

ISBN 0–8039–8198–8

Library of Congress Catalog card number 88–63020

Typeset by Photoprint, Torquay, Devon
Printed in Great Britain by J.W. Arrowsmith Ltd, Bristol

Contents

1 Problems of Organizational Rationality in Health Systems:
  Political Controls and Policy Options   1
  Giorgio Freddi

2 Politicizing Medicine and Medicalizing Politics:
  Physician Power in the United States   28
  James Warner Björkman

3 Health Professionals in the Swedish System   74
  Jan-Erik Lane and Sven Arvidson

4 Controlling Dutch Health Care   99
  *Nico Baakman, Jan van der Made
  and Ingrid Mur-Veeman*

5 The Politics of Health Reform: Origins and Performance
  of the Italian Health Service in Comparative Perspective   116
  Maurizio Ferrera

6 Physicians and the State in France   130
  David Wilsford

7 Hospital Planners and Medical Professionals in the
  Federal Republic of Germany   157
  Christa Altenstetter

8 Physicians' Professional Autonomy in the Welfare State:
  Endangered or Preserved?   178
  Marian Döhler

9 Clinical Autonomy in the United Kingdom and the
  United States: Contrasts and Convergence   198
  Stephen Harrison and Rockwell I. Schulz

10 Structure and Performance of the Medical Care Delivery
   Systems of the United Kingdom and the United States   210
   J. Rogers Hollingsworth

   References   230
   Index   245
   Notes on the Contributors   249

Preface

At the 1985 Joint Sessions of Workshops of the European Consortium for Political Research, some twenty scholars convened in Barcelona at a workshop on the politics of health. All the chapters in this volume (other than the first and the sixth) were originally presented at the workshop, but each has subsequently been thoroughly revised and rewritten. Since constraints of space prevented the inclusion of every paper presented in Barcelona, the editors chose to select those national case studies and comparative materials that illuminate the universal problem of governing the health sector in modern politics. Nonetheless, editing proved to be a difficult task when editors as well as authors kept moving among the continents of Europe, Asia and North America. The editors thank the authors for patiently accepting editorial directives and only regret the relentless creep of time that delayed publication beyond initial expectations. Fortunately the contents of this volume are not narrowly time-bound, and so its generalizations remain valid in the sometimes seemingly kaleidoscopic world of national health policies and the politics which envelop them.

Giorgio Freddi
Bologna, Italy

James Warner Björkman
Hyderabad, India

1

Problems of Organizational Rationality in Health Systems: Political Controls and Policy Options

Giorgio Freddi

Governmental Intervention in the Health Sector and Medical Autonomy: the Background

All Western political systems are characterized by governmental intervention in the delivery of medical services. The reasons why governments began to intervene, the modes of their interventions, and the moments in history when intervention was initiated vary greatly from country to country. However, all the political systems are now confronted – and have been for several decades – with a common predicament which has caused and is causing governmental intervention to become more intense, penetrating, and oriented towards control of performance. Three factors can be distinguished in this more recent development, of which two are specific and one is of a more general nature.

In the first place a highly sophisticated and technological medicine (both diagnostic and therapeutic) has emerged which, though relatively effective, is at the same time exceedingly costly. Secondly, and more or less simultaneously, larger and larger numbers of citizens have gained access to these new kinds of medical care and treatment; this, in turn, has everywhere driven the health bill to consume unprecedented percentages of the GNP. Finally, the increase in health-related expenditures has taken place in the context of the fiscal crisis of the welfare state, thus reinforcing governmental motivations to monitor medical services delivery systems and to introduce more stringent control procedures.

The combined effects of both earlier interventions into the health sector – largely prompted by political and ideological considerations – and more recent and pragmatic attempts to contain costs have induced the rise of huge public health structures. Now medical services are delivered in a highly institutionalized environment.

Three characteristics of this environment are singled out for discussion in this chapter. The first is its proximity to the political system. The second is its complexity. The third is the fact that doctors, once the (almost) sole decision-makers, vested with an authority verging on charisma, must now share their power with a host of other actors; bureaucrats, politicians, trade unions, consumer groups, and fiscal intermediaries constitute a singularly intricate network of constraints encompassing and encroaching on the doctors' specific domain. More precisely, this chapter is concerned with the comparative analysis of how the expansion, politicization, and complexity of the public health sector have affected the traditional autonomy of its central actors, the doctors, and of the new patterns which seem to be emerging.

Such an analysis involves the investigation of two closely intertwined dimensions of a very sensitive policy area, or what we might call the external and the internal spheres of the public health complex. On the one hand are the contextual conditions (ideological, cultural, institutional) which describe and explain modes of intervention in the health arena; and on the other hand are the institutional and stylistic contexts that illuminate and denote the redistribution of decisional power in the medical services delivery systems following public intervention.

As shown in the other chapters of this book and in the voluminous and rapidly growing international literature on the subject, public health arrangements for the organization and operations of the health sector differ greatly from one country to another. This diversity might appear somewhat surprising because we are dealing with a policy space characterized by outwardly quite common properties, at least among Western nations: the tradition of scientific inquiry, the training and ethic of the medical profession, and a widely shared technology, all would lead us to expect conditions of uniformity rather than heterogeneity. Moreover, contextual and environmental circumstances would be expected to encourage homogeneity as all our national referents fall into the genus of the economically developed, highly industrialized, urban societies governed by democratic, representative, and pluralist political institutions. Yet, when we contemplate national modes of public intervention in the health domain, and the ways in which such modes impinge on medical autonomy, we face a bewildering array of organizational schemes and of functional and behavioural patterns. Indeed, if a common unifying rationality were to be sought, none – most probably – would be found.

The Need for a Comparative Taxonomy

Ideally one should strive toward constructing a typology capable of ordering, relating, and eventually explaining the phenomena and issues summarized in the preceding section. Here, however, I shall be content to make a first step in that direction by proposing a taxonomic framework to be employed for comparative exercises, which draws from paradigms and models developed and articulated in the disciplinary fields of public policy analysis and organization theory.

The dependent variable of such a framework is medical professional autonomy. The taxonomy aims to identify independent variables: that is, those factors – capable of being analysed comparatively – that condition both the direction in which and the extent to which medical autonomy has, or has not, been modified in a number of Western political systems. The empirical referents for comparison are discussed in subsequent chapters of this volume.

The independent variables can be grouped according to two main comprehensive categories:

1 The political environment of the public health complex and its influence on institutional arrangements and policy predispositions
2 The institutional environment of the public health complex, particularly the type of organizational rationality prevailing in and characterizing medical services delivery systems.

Before discussing these two sets of independent variables, careful attention should be devoted to the construction of a critical and analytical definition of the notion of medical professional autonomy. At least two excellent reasons exist for doing so. First, the notion is frequently used in such a way as to make its meaning ambiguous and internally contradictory. Secondly, the notion itself has undergone substantive changes stemming from evolutionary trends that have everywhere affected the practice of medicine and the delivery of medical services. In fact, as will be seen, it is because of these changes that ambiguity and internal contradictions now plague the notion of medical autonomy.

Medical Autonomy: from the Soloist to the Orchestra

The notion of medical autonomy is closely related to that of medical professionalism, as has been made clear in a recent critical review

(Björkman 1982) of the literature on the professions specifically concerned with the practice of medicine. In other words, autonomy is portrayed as an indispensable hallmark of professionalization (Moore 1970). Let us see briefly how this has worked to transform the craft of the healer into the profession of the medical man.

An occupation evolves into a community of professionals when, in the practice of that occupation, decisions are based on an esoteric, academic, highly technical knowledge and on a common ethic which stresses both the interests of clients and a service orientation. Moreover, the professional community indemnifies the public by controlling the recruitment, selection, and training of its members, and by exercising disciplinary power over those members who trespass the boundaries of legitimate and technically warranted professional action.

Autonomy, however, does not follow automatically from the demonstrable existence and viability of the above requisites. Rather, autonomy is something which is granted to a profession by society and specifically by the state. Inevitably this step involves, among other things, the profession itself in the political process. Such societal and governmental sanction implies that the professional community has acquired a quality of elitist authoritativeness which deserves protection from outside encroachments on both its right to self-government and its decisional and operational standards. In our case it implies that the medical profession enjoys a monopolistic control over the knowledge and definition of ill health and its treatment, and that its members have been and are being so thoroughly socialized as to make it extremely improbable that they will not behave stringently in accordance with professional ethic and techniques. Incidentally, such deductive logic ought not to imply that these definitional propositions always pass the empirical test, as has been shown by several studies (Björkman 1982). However, evidence that physicians sometimes misbehave, and that the profession not infrequently fails to discipline them, does not affect the thrust of my arguments.

At this very general level, the definitions just set forth capture the quintessence of the medical profession and persuasively explain why it has been granted autonomy. However, as soon as we analyse the operational criteria whereby the medical profession can be taken to be autonomous – as soon as we single out the functional components of autonomy – we face heuristic ambiguities and contradictions. The main reason is that both the academic and the political debates about medical autonomy are, to varying degrees, still side-tracked by an interpretation which, while empirically grounded at a time when medicine was a 'liberal' profession, is no longer supported by fact. To a remarkable extent, what used to be a sound description of the real world of medical practice now increasingly resembles ideology. I submit that the structures and behavioural patterns which embodied the notion of medical autonomy until roughly four decades ago have undergone an evolutionary transformation that has changed them almost beyond recognition.

Let us see why and how by analysing a catalogue of the requisites for autonomy. Scholars who have attempted empirical research in this field (Harrison et al. 1984) report that doctors themselves have difficulties in articulating a clear-cut definition of their autonomy, but the following list obtains a relatively broad consensus:

1 The remuneration of physicians according to the fee-for-service formula, whereby fees are paid directly by patients to doctors and are freely determined by the latter
2 The right to independent practice, that is clinical autonomy, connoted by the sanctity of a highly individualized doctor–patient relationship, which ensures that diagnostic and therapeutic decisions are subject to no external control
3 The responsibility to lead and coordinate other health professionals (Tolliday 1978)
4 The processing of professional issues according to a social consensus model of behaviour which excludes the conflict-based processes inherent in unionization (Krause 1977).

Even a cursory examination of the situations now obtaining in Western political systems shows that none of these four criteria has gone unscathed. Indeed, in some national cases they have been virtually obliterated, and everywhere they have been greatly diluted. Naturally there are differences in the degree of dilution from country to country, so that the criteria for autonomy can be conceptualized as continua along which differences can be assessed in terms of the independent variables discussed in the following sections. Here I sketch out how the evolutionary changes of the last 40 years have affected our four criteria.

Remuneration
The first criterion, the manner of remuneration of doctors, has been most palpably affected. The fee-for-service arrangement has been the first line of defence against public intervention in the health care sector. The physicians' guilds have given it the highest symbolic significance as the bastion that, once demolished, would allow outside controls over clinical practice and a deterioration of the quality of medical services. Yet the fee-for-service scheme is now

largely a relic of the past. Doctors are being remunerated in a number of ways; these can be ordered along a continuum which, in turn, tends to be correlated with the degree of 'organizational density' (as Döhler phrases it in chapter 8) of public intervention. The sequence in the continuum from most flexible to least flexible arrangements can be expressed as: fee for service; payments through private insurance carriers without ceilings for the amounts charged; the same method with specified ceilings for types of treatment; public or semi-public insurance schemes; salary schedules that allow for individual merit increases; salary schedules linked to a combination of rank and seniority; and capitation.

Doctors have opposed the demise of the fee-for-service arrangement for several (understandable) reasons. First, even the mildest form of fiscal intermediation potentially introduces the possibility of income control and eventually of income reduction – even though (as Björkman clearly demonstrates in chapter 2), under certain conditions observed in the US, fiscal intermediation can bring about income increases. Secondly, almost any kind of fiscal intermediation, let alone salary schedules and capitation, involves a loss of social prestige: the traditional professional man is paid an honorarium which manifestly is a very elitist manner of remuneration.

Thirdly, physicians have consistently and adamantly maintained that the growth of an institutionalized health complex inevitably leads to a restriction of professional (clinical) autonomy and to a subsequent reduction of the quality of services. In fact, this position is still an article of faith universally proclaimed by the medical guilds. In chapter 8 Döhler argues cogently that these contentions are not factually grounded. On the contrary, empirical findings show little or no relation between the loss of an autonomous income and a degradation of clinical autonomy. In sum, public organizational density and professional autonomy do not seem to be interdependent dimensions. Döhler's argument rests on the classic and authoritative definition of clinical autonomy and, against that background, is very forceful. We will, nevertheless, see that if we adopt a more evolutionary view of clinical autonomy; a significant relationship between organizational density and the modes of clinical autonomy can be observed.

Independent practice

Our second criterion is specifically concerned with the hard core of medical ideology, that is, with clinical autonomy defined as 'the ability of the physician to make autonomous decisions concerning the contents and the conditions of the medical working process' (Freidson 1973: 368). Literally interpreted, this definition can be applied only to a past age of professional practice, when most medical services were delivered by individual practitioners. Indeed, as Harrison and Schulz point out in chapter 9,

> This idealized picture [of the independent practitioner] was never wholly accurate since there were always some third parties in the form of hospital owners, friendly societies and the like; but it clearly differed from present-day reality . . . third parties are now entrenched actors in every health care system in the world . . . It is the increasing importance of these third parties which makes clinical autonomy into an issue, for it raises questions about the extent to which professionals are (or should be) free from controls by them.

This quotation again focuses on the problem of organizational density and, more generally, on the machinery of the welfare state, for the single greatest influence behind the increase of organizational density is attributed to public intervention. Moreover it calls attention to the fact that nowadays the great majority of physicians operate in highly structured organizational environments.

At this juncture, however, another crucial item must be injected into the discussion. The principal reason that doctors work in organizations – with all the constraints on individual behaviour ensuing therefrom – is to be found not so much in economic and/or political developments as in the very complexity of contemporary medicine. The delivery of medical services requires highly sophisticated teamwork that calls for equally sophisticated structures through which the myriad of new medical specialties and allied technologies and professions are coordinated. Even the term *gatekeeper*, which has been appropriated to denote the present role of the traditional general practitioner, is suggestive of a systemic environment, of an intricate network of interdependencies. This situation goes far beyond the problem of intraprofessional relationships (Larkin 1983). The organizations that constitute the environment for medical action may be hierarchically skewed and centralized or they may be loosely coupled flat structures, but the field is characterized by the usual arsenal of specialization, hierarchy, division of labour, control, and so forth. In fact, quite some time ago, Coser (1958) cogently observed that in medical activities, the higher the technology and more complex the team, the greater is the probability of finding hierarchically structured situations.

Viewed in this light, the issue of autonomy acquires different contours. It is not primarily a question of protecting the individual physician from institutional encroachment but rather – as the classic literature (Marcson 1960; Kornhauser 1962) about professionals in organizations has maintained for a long time – one of insuring those organizational conditions which allow for the correct deployment of professional decisional and operational standards.

Leadership

The third criterion posits a strong correlation between the safeguard of autonomy and the medical personnel's responsibility to lead and coordinate other health professionals. Here too we detect a flavour of remembrance of things past: there has been a major shift from the strong hierarchical role that the physician played some 30–40 years ago, to one in which he is required to share power for decision-making with paramedics and with other technology-oriented health professionals. The latter now have a larger share of responsibility for patient care, a share that has increased at the expense of the physician's share (Perkoff 1984).

The recently emerged self-awareness and militancy of the other health professions only partially elucidate why doctors lost much of their power. The central condition for change is represented here too by the organizational and technological complexity of contemporary health care: the physician alone simply can no longer cope with the new task domains. This is particularly true when we focus on the most complex of health organizations, the hospital. The history of the modern hospital is the history of the steady decline of the physician's hierarchic power to control his work environment.

The revolutionary technological and scientific advances of health care which took place at the outset of this century caused the power of control to shift from the boards of trustees to the great clinicians and surgeons who were able to manage the hospital competently. For approximately the first half of this century, the medical elite's power was authoritarian and absolute; it extended its reach to all personnel, ranging from junior doctors, 'ancillary' specialists and other health professionals, to administrative and menial staff. Yet confronted by events since 1950, the medical elite has been unable to retain its exalted role. There is no medical craftsman, no matter how good, who can successfully cope with such disparate and mutually reinforcing factors as the increasing complexity of in-patient care and diagnostic medicine; the proliferation of specialists; the dominant role played by hospitals in organizing and servicing community health programmes; preventive medicine; and all this in a context characterized by the democratization of endo-organizational relationships.

These radical innovations, plus the establishment of a close relationship between hospital and community – which led to the rise of a more or less loosely coupled health system involving nearly all health actors within and without the hospital – have emphasized the need for a new type of institutional leader. Such a leader must, at one and the same time, be knowledgeable about medical techniques, well versed in management, and adept at political processes (Perrow 1961, 1963; Perkoff 1979). The result is visible, in varying measures, in all Western nations: a rapid growing professionalization of administrators who interpret dominant coordinative roles.

At this point it must be stressed that the expansion of the welfare state and the concomitant mass access to complex and sophisticated medical care have compounded the phenomenon, but not created it. The trend is inherent in the fundamental changes of medical services delivery. It seems fair, then, to conclude that the physician, who used to be a soloist, has become the member of an orchestra whose conductor, moreover, is not necessarily a physician. As was noted with respect to our second criterion, the problem remains to assess whether, in different political systems, this new situation has been tackled in a manner safeguarding professional modes of action.

Control of the profession

According to our fourth and last criterion, the protection of professional autonomy is also contingent upon the ability of doctors' guilds to exhibit a social consensus model of behaviour and correlatively to avoid conflict-based action. A quick comparative perusal of Western societies makes plain that this criterion too has been eroded, in many instances beyond repair. Recent events are largely responsible for this erosion, together with the socio-cultural characteristics of the medical associations of different countries. For both environmental and structural reasons, the doctors' guilds were born and/or grew weaker or stronger in various political systems (Martinelli 1983), with the result that some have been better equipped than others to withstand recent onslaughts on professional autonomy. In fact, if we distribute along a continuum of decreasing associational autonomy the medical communities active in the Western world, we can distinguish between classic professional associations; monolithic neo-corporatist bodies; cohesive unions, and union fragmentation.

I now turn to a comparative discussion of the four criteria analysed so far, in the light of the two sets of independent variables presented earlier.

Cultures, Policy Predispositions,
and Institutional Contexts

So far I have argued that the comparative assessment of medical autonomy – no longer guaranteed by individual and independent practice – is predominantly a function of the organizational structures which necessarily constitute the environment of contemporary medicine. However, the character and articulation of such organizational structures vary in different countries and thus may be more or less congruent with the requisites for professional action.

To develop a comparative framework for a comprehensive investigation or organizational variations and their impact on medical professionalism I propose to discuss and interpret institutional differences in the light of policy predispositions and policy styles (Richardson 1982) as affected by broader and overarching cultural conditions.

A very forceful conceptual tool for the comparative analysis of policy styles and predispositions is that fashioned by Douglas and Wildavsky (1982) and later persuasively put through the empirical test by Wildavsky (1986). These authors begin by constructing pure ideal types of cultural orientation, which they label and define as follows.

Competitive individualism is a market culture. Its only rule is that limits on transactions should be restricted to the protection of people and property; the promise of market cultures is that 'they will continuously generate greater resources so that all involved will be better (though not equally well) off' (Wildavsky 1986: 30). Socio-economic processes are 'fair to individualists who have opportunities to enter and benefit from competition' (1986: 30). The ethos of this cultural type is best expressed by equality of opportunity.

Hierarchical collectivism is the cultural orientation typical of strongly bounded collectives. In a hierarchical collective, 'fairness follows function' (1986: 32); being fairly treated does not mean being treated like everyone else, but being treated according to one's status and predictable rules. The main concern, then, is with legal equality.

Sectarianism is a cultural mode applying to collectives that are strongly bounded but have an absolute minimum of rules, with voluntary action playing a dominant role and authority relationships ideally non-existent. No one is to have more of anything, especially power, than anyone else, yet everyone must agree. Equality of condition (and of results) is emphasized, for, without authority, this is the only way in which individuals can relate to one another.

Thus, individualism is associated with equality of opportunity, collectivism with legal equality, and sectarianism with equality of results. To quote again Aaron Wildavsky:

> Though everyone speaks approvingly of equality, each means something different. There is a world of difference between equality of opportunity, to be different, equality of results, to be the same, and equality before the law, to legitimate differences. Whether policies are designed to diminish or decrease differences among people is a telltale sign of which political culture is preferred. (1986: 33)

As we have learned from Max Weber, there are no ideal types to be seen in the real world. There, we find hybrid types; actual situations and patterns combine the properties of ideal types in different proportions. Consequently, if we seek those hybrid types which may be constructed by observing the trends consolidated in the countries studied in this volume, three basic cultural patterns emerge.

Europe may be characterized as having very strong collectivism, moderate individualism, and social democratic moderate sects. Most European political systems share a historical development marked by a strong sense of sovereignty and by an extremely hierarchical bureaucratic tradition (Freddi 1982, 1986). As we shall see, however, two partially different cultural configurations are discernible within Europe according to whether the emphasis is placed on legal equality – generally associated with a prevalence of moderate and/or conservative forces in the political arena – or on a more sectarian equality of results, which tends to be evident in stabilized social democracies or in peculiar situations such as that which can be observed in Italy.

On the other hand, the political culture of the US may be considered as combining weak collectivism (due to the lack of a hierarchical tradition), strong individualism, and quite an active streak of sectarianism. A mere glance at American history shows why sectarianism is so much in evidence. The US was largely settled by Protestant sects that brought with them a deep mistrust of state power; indeed the American Revolution was fought against executive power. A weak state, still to be regarded with suspicion as the very source of hierarchical inequality, became then a permanent hallmark of the American polity

During most of the nineteenth century there were moderate contrasts between the sectarian and the competitive individualistic orientations; that is, while there were disagreements between sects and markets over the extent of allowable inequality, these were held in check. As long as the government was weak, markets seemed to create the best conditions for the achievement of true equality.

> Once inequality was laid at the door of central government, moreover, competitive individualism could be reconciled with egalitarian sectarianism – equality of opportunity with equality of result – by claiming that an attack on authority (i.e. central government) could increase equality of opportunity, which would then, once artificial fetters were removed, naturally lead to equality of result. (Wildavsky 1986: 38)

It was with the rise of the giant corporation that this happy coincidence of the orientations shaping American political culture came to an end. Monopolies soon came to be perceived as hierarchies leading to more and more inequality. The sectarian component, though continuing to mistrust authority, then began advocating greater governmental intervention.

Using the Douglas and Wildavsky paradigm as a system of coordinates, a series of comparisons can be drawn between the US and Europe and among European countries to illustrate the range of developments in the area of health-related public policies.

After the completion of the Industrial Revolution, as inequality grew more and more visible, the social and political movements advocating equality of result – our sectarians – were faced with a radical alternative. Either they could give up on equality and adapt to the life of individualism, as the American sectarians did by moving toward the dominant culture of competitive capitalism; or they could accept authority by adopting hierarchical modes of action and organization as the European sectarians did, who were confronted with worse conditions of inequality than in the US.

This chain of events is at the origin of the great divide we now observe between the American and the European approaches to public intervention. In Europe, after the national processes of political development had been fulfilled and mass democracies had been established, that is when the notion of *political citizenship* became entrenched and the road leading to the welfare state was being gradually and slowly opened, the notion of *social citizenship* was created to give legitimacy and ideological dignity to public intervention (Eisenstadt and Rokkan 1973). Thus, as the degree of social differentiation increased and the probability that markets could be able to satisfy an optimal, or merely acceptable, combination of interests and expectations correspondingly decreased, organized pressures for public intervention mounted (Lehner and Widmaier 1983). By contrast the US remains anchored to the notion of political citizenship as the main legitimating criterion of the polity and its social benefits.

The answers to social demands have consistently diverged in the US and in Europe. The clear trend in Europe favours solidarity coupled with equality, whereas the US retains market efficiency coupled with liberty. Coherently with these premises, social policies in many European systems have tended to take the form of provisions of services in kind or of merit goods. On the contrary, in the US preference has been consistently accorded to cash transfers aimed at the goal of income maintenance. In the former case, the main thrust has been towards universalism wherein all citizens benefit equally from social policies regardless of income; the overarching methods have favoured institutional redistribution (Titmuss 1974) and social justice. In the American case, policies favour a particularistic approach through which only the needy receive help; in so doing, an equilibrium based on equality of opportunity is re-established and the individuals thus benefited are encouraged to re-enter the market.

As noted above, in Europe there are differences of style and orientation among different political systems that, while more or less homogeneously characterized by hierarchical collectivism, differ in the degree to which they exhibit egalitarian (sectarian) propensities. Policy predispositions partial to equality of result tend to be in evidence in those countries where left-wing parties (mostly of the social democratic persuasion) have been in power over a long period (as in Sweden and England) or at least have been in a strategically influential position (as the Italian Communist Party) when important legislation concerning medical services delivery was being considered and enacted. Sweden, England and Italy, in fact, are the three countries that have opted for a policy of provision of services in kind by instituting national health services.

The opposite seems to apply where moderate and/or conservative governments have exerted much sway in shaping social policies. The semi-public insurance scheme is the basic vehicle for the delivery of medical services in the French, Dutch, and German cases. In Germany this has continued to be true also during and after a long period marked by social democratic majorities – which might be seen as contradicting our generalization. However, limits to the collectivization of social services and to the unlimited expansion of social rights seem to be systemic in the Federal Republic, where the principle of the 'social market', positing an interdependent connection between the extent and continuity of social rights and a sustained economic growth, has received constitutional sanction (Scase 1977; Ginsburg 1979).

Against the background of cultural and institutional factors considered in the preceding paragraphs, let us now see how the public health programmes operating in the countries discussed in this volume have affected the status and autonomy of physicians, and how much damage has been inflicted on the once elitist stance of the medical profession. In Europe two medical systems – the German and the Dutch – have retained classic autonomy to a remarkable extent, while the others – Britain, France, Sweden, and Italy – have experienced serious assaults on autonomy, even if of a different intensity and quality.

West Germany

In the Federal Republic the policy environment is distinguished by the original arrangement of German federalism. The central government is engaged in the larger questions of policy while the *Länder* do most of the work concerned with regulation and implementation. At the local level, moreover, regulatory actions by the government do not have an authoritative bent; on the contrary, one observes a high measure of interest-group integration, with a preferred reliance on negotiation among groups rather than an imposition of arbitrary and binding decisions. Regulation, in public health policy as well as in other policy domains, constitutes the fundamental feature of the German style (Dyson 1982). Regulations are formulated and implemented in a manner that is best described as corporatist.

The central conditions for corporatism are almost perfectly exhibited by the character and action patterns of the regional medical associations. These are cohesive and disciplined, and their appointed leaders can speak confidently for the entire profession, without fear of being contradicted and/or weakened by internecine conflict. When they negotiate economic transactions with the equally autonomous and corporatist sickness funds, or when they bargain with public authorities over annual increases of health expenditures (see Döhler in chapter 8), they act with one voice. Everyone else concerned knows that they represent the profession and by and large can guarantee its behaviour.

The outcomes of these thorough negotiations in Germany are made even more reliable and predictable by the style of administration and implementation displayed by the *ad hoc* regional agencies (see Altenstetter in chapter 7). Here, the very cohesive cultural dimension of hierarchical collectivism married to corporatism is further cemented by the great normative power of legal forms (Eckstein 1979) typical of the German governmental tradition. Thus a political-administrative structure which stresses legal tradition, normativism, and formalism gives the medical profession extraordinary leeway for its continued dominance over health care processes (see chapter 7).

The Netherlands
The Dutch case is also marked by a signal incidence of corporatist arrangements, to a degree even higher than that observed in Germany. As Baakman, van der Made, and Mur-Veeman have meticulously documented in chapter 4, Dutch physicians are protected against state encroachment on their professional activities by a truly exceptional collection of safeguards. Several factors account for this state of affairs, among which the following are the most striking:

1 Regulations regarding health policy and institutions in the Netherlands are formulated by a number of consultative and/or decisional bodies (Council of Hospital Facilities, National Health Council, Central Organization for Health Tariffs, and Sickness Funds Council) representing the various actors of the health policy establishment that all belong in the family of quasi non-governmental organizations (quangos), thus keeping doctors at a safe distance from governmental institutions.
2 In all these bodies the number of seats assigned to physicians and hospital representatives constitutes the majority in some instances, nearly always a plurality, of the total.
3 Measures passed allegedly to control physicians' professional behaviour *de facto* have more the status of recommendations than of authoritative rulings.

While in Germany the corporatist pattern of organic integration of the doctors into the health policy process is buttressed by a normative and legalistic policy establishment, in the Netherlands the already formidable power held by the physicians' guild is further strengthened by the consociational structure of the polity. For instance, hospitals and other health-related institutions – let alone sickness funds – can be catalogued according to the tripartite breakdown of Dutch subcultures (Protestant, Catholic and secular), so that advice and decisions issuing from the health quangos hardly run the risk of encountering really dangerous opposition from either central or local public authorities. To sum up the Dutch experience, nowhere in the Western world is the classic definition of medical autonomy translated into practice more accurately than in the Netherlands.

France
Quite a different picture is to be seen in the other four European cases. Viewed from the fiscal and organizational configuration of

the public health system, France, whose medical services delivery system is articulated on semi-public insurance schemes, should be classified in the same category as Germany and the Netherlands. Yet with regard to medical autonomy, the French case has very little to share with these two countries.

Three interdependent ingredients affect the French case in a very distinct manner. In the first place, while France assuredly shares the cultural dimension of hierarchical collectivism, it emphasizes the symbolic component of a centralized version of sovereignty and the functional component of *étatisme*; by and large the state is expected to take the initiative in setting social-economic policies. Consequently the French civil service, especially the senior staff, views itself as an elite corps guarding the general interest and embodying state sovereignty. In sum, the state apparatus is ill-disposed toward negotiation with interest groups.

Secondly, France is not a pluralist political society. While voluntary associations exist in France in abundance, pluralism is not sanctioned in the official ideology of the French state. In some polities pluralism is perceived as a positive value, and encouraged to expand; in others – signally in France – the opposite applies. There it is perceived as a selfishly particularistic form of action, inherently hostile and harmful to the general interest. As Wilsford points out in chapter 6, one of the oldest laws (*loi* Le Chapelier) of the republic, dating to the Revolution of 1789, allows voluntary associations to exist only by sufferance, and with great circumspection at that. This explains why medical associations were never a significant force in France: more clearly than elsewhere, medical autonomy has always been construed as a privilege that, having been granted by the state, could accordingly be taken away.

Finally, French political culture is fragmented. Interest groups' activities and programmes tend to be blurred and made imprecise and internally contradictory by deep-seated ideological issues. The consequences of associational weakness and fragmentation are evident. Instead of a single medical guild in France, there is a myriad of doctors' unions – an indicator of lack of autonomy, as we have seen. These unions are frequently antagonistic among themselves and constantly in conflict with the central government (see Wilsford in chapter 6, and Döhler in chapter 8).

Even though there are provisions for consultation between physicians' representatives and the bureaucracy, for the most part such consultations end up being frustrating exercises. The frequent recourse to strikes is an indication of the impotence of doctors *vis-à-vis* the administration (see chapter 6), as are episodes of uncommonly heavy-handed intervention of the state in the most jealous prerogatives of the medical profession such as training, internal governance, and the setting of technical standards (Jamous 1969). To sum up, French medicine could very well be described as administered medicine. It is a profession with a very limited capacity to define and control its work environment.

United Kingdom
Britain is the first Western nation to have introduced a universalistic public health programme based on the provision of services in kind, the National Health Service. The egalitarian principles that connote the delivery of medical services to the public has a harmonious counterpart in the manner of remuneration of physicians. The general practitioners, or gatekeepers, are remunerated according to the capitation method. Specialists and hospital physicians have been accorded a status akin to that of the civil servants; they receive salaries, but there is some leeway in the system for merit increases.

The physicians' guilds are cohesive and well organized and, in the British policy style (Jordan and Richardson 1982), are involved in closed consultations and negotiations with the bureaucracy to determine periodic upgradings of remunerations (see Döhler in chapter 8, and Harrison and Schulz in chapter 9). Since the inception of the NHS, the government's main concern has been that of containing the budget, which it has done successfully; funds are allocated to semi-autonomous health authorities, with a minimum of operational guidelines from central administration. Within these tight budget constraints, physicians act largely unhampered by managerial controls. In fact, there is a governmental guarantee of clinical freedom expressly stated in the original legislation instituting the NHS. As a consequence, a consensus exists that management is a process of facilitating the work of professionals rather than exerting control over them (see chapter 9). Nevertheless, this seems to be a rather attenuated version of clinical autonomy. Physicians are – so to speak – left to their own devices as long as they do not trespass into the policy-making and managerial arenas. British medical services delivery is in fact highly bureaucratized, with visibly negative consequences for its ability to innovate and upgrade the doctors' trade (see Hollingsworth in chapter 10).

Sweden
The Swedish policy style accentuates 'an activist role for the state that involves some blurring of the distinction between public and private interests' (Kelman 1981: 338–9). One is not surprised, then, to find quite a streak of egalitarian sectarianism in the public health sector. During the last twenty years, as Lane and Arvidson

relate in chapter 3, Sweden has gradually shifted from a medical services delivery system articulated on a number of insurance schemes with central government guidance and support, to a national health service whose management and financing is almost entirely decentralized to the county councils and the largest municipal governments.

Physicians have correspondingly experienced a notable change in their status and in their ability to control the work environment. They have moved from an institutional setup characterized by relatively mild bureaucratic controls from the centre, to a quite different one where doctors are engaged in face-to-face relationships with the political personnel of local governments; from a situation where their income was partially a function of private practice to a comprehensive salaried status; from an actual control of the work environment via the power of supervision over other health professionals, to a more formally structured system of coordination of the various professions and specialties run by professional managers. Moreover, their guild no longer exhibits the traits of a professional association, but rather shows those usually found in a trade union – as the increasing resort to strikes makes obvious.

It is not surprising, therefore, that Swedish doctors' relationships with the other health professions and occupations are strained. When they seek to introduce changes or innovative measures, they can count on having a difficult time with the county councils and on meeting with the hostility of the other health-related unions.

Swedish medicine has been on the defensive for the last twenty years and has lost many of the prerogatives that gave it an authoritative posture in policy-making and in controlling the work environment (Carder and Klingeberg 1980). However, in the very narrow interpretation that has been seen to apply to the English case, clinical autonomy has been preserved in Sweden too.

Italy

Italy introduced a national health service, the Servizio Sanitario Nazionale (SSN), in 1978, replacing a health system articulated on a multitude of semi-public insurance schemes. As Ferrera argues in chapter 5, to comprehend fully the impact of this reform on medical autonomy, the political conditions obtaining at the time when the reform was enacted must be investigated. It was then that the political coalition which the late secretary of the Communist Party, Enrico Berlinguer, had advocated under the celebrated label of 'historic compromise' took concrete form (Pasquino 1987: 228–34). From 1976 to 1979 Italy was governed by a cabinet of 'national solidarity' supported in Parliament by the centrist and centre-left parties, as well as the Communists, who had actively participated in the formulation of the governmental programme.

The rationale behind such a large coalition was that a cabinet of national solidarity was needed to tackle an emergency situation successfully. Economic recession, mounting unemployment, terrorism, and highly mobilized movements within the trade unions and among students called for stern measures that needed a very broad legitimation.

The SSN is the most representative brainchild of this experiment. As such, it inevitably exhibits a mix of contradictory and extreme traits. Not only did the SSN embody the sometimes reciprocally incongruent ideological and programmatic predilections of so many and oddly assorted coalition partners, but also the political parties supporting the government tried to defuse potentially explosive issues heralded by the trade unions and the student movement by introducing radically egalitarian (sectarian) measures in the new public health system. The SSN became the structural vehicle not only of symbolic values demonstrably and directly related to a wide-reaching programme of public health – such as the idea that free medical assistance is but an extension of the notion of democratic citizenship – but also of other symbols and values whose political relevance is not in doubt, but which evidence no direct relationship with the public delivery of medical services (Freddi 1984a). A brief synopsis follows of these value premises and of the structural arrangements that have been designed to accommodate them.

Democratic decentralization The SSN is now the responsibility of regional governments that receive nearly all their finances from the central treasury. Regional governments, however, act as cashiers and controllers of expenditure, while the actual delivery of medical services has been assigned to 600 *unità sanitarie locali* (USL) or local health units. These finance, manage, direct, control and coordinate all health-related structures and personnel operating in their territorial jurisdictions.

Democratic participation in management The top management functions of each USL are performed by so-called managing committees or *comitati di gestione*, whose members are elected by the municipal councils whose territorial jurisdictions fall into that of the USL. They are served by administrative and technical staffs.

Populist sectarianism The members of the USL's managing committees are elected by municipal councils *from their own memberships*. On the whole they tend to be small-time politicians if not downright political jobbers. Even though they administer budgets of an order of magnitude comparable with those of medium and sometimes large corporations, and manage technologically sophisticated structures and personnel, no previous training or experience even remotely related to the health sector is required of them (DeSantis and Ferrera 1983; Freddi 1984a). Findings from these studies also show, however, that the members of managing committees represent all political parties roughly in proportion to the latter's electoral strength. A climate of sectarian populism prevails here which entails an unadulterated spoils system based on the notion that 'anybody can do it'.

Anti-technocratic and anti-elitist bias   Throughout the SSN, physicians are systematically cut off from policy formulation and management; they are excluded from any and all relevant authority relationships. The classic criteria for medical autonomy hardly apply any longer. General practitioners are remunerated according to the capitation method, while rigid bureaucratic constraints on their clinical autonomy have been introduced. Hospital physicians' career patterns are strictly modelled after civil service rules, with seniority as the main standard for promotions. They are allowed a minimum of private practice within the hospital. Hospital medical personnel, however, can opt for a part-time solution, and those who choose to do so have some opportunities for additional income. However, while the private sector has grown increasingly prosperous, doctors face very strong competition as the ratio of physicians to the population is by far the highest in the Western world – one doctor per 284 inhabitants (Bompiani 1984: 151) compared with one per 350 to 700 inhabitants in other European systems.

All in all, Italian physicians who choose to work inside the SSN must function within a constrained interpretation of autonomy. They have no control over the work environment which – as has been seen – is extremely politicized. Those who are ambitious and wish to develop specific programmes must involve themselves deeply in politics. We might say, then, that the dominant role played by the central bureaucracy in France is, in Italy, being played by the party system (Freddi 1984a). No wonder, then, that there are about twenty medical unions, which can be classified by the simultaneous application of the three criteria of medical specialty, rank and seniority of the membership, and ideological persuasion. And less wonder still that they resort to strikes as the normal approach to negotiation, most of the time independently of one another.

United States
As we follow the fascinating narrative of the case of the US given by Björkman (chapter 2), we cannot but conclude that we are looking

here at another instance of American exceptionalism. There is no doubt that, since the inception of Medicaid and Medicare, and after the government's repeated interventions aimed at making those programmes economically viable, medical autonomy is no longer what it used to be. Indeed, if we accept the conventional stipulation whereby clinical autonomy is the function of individual independence, we must conclude that there has been a radical change (in addition to chapter 2, see also chapters 8 and 9). Yet, if we compare the modes of American public intervention in the health sector and the institutional outcomes of that intervention with the European cases that have been discussed above, the contrast could not be more striking. The two basic European approaches to intervention (corporatist negotiation and direct administration) are nowhere to be seen in the US.

On the one hand the close consultation between interest groups and governmental agencies, which represents the norm in some European cases where collectivism is so strong, would be impossible in the US. Seen in terms of the sectarian dimension of American culture, consultation would be suspect, possibly illicit, even tantamount to conspiracy. On the other hand, stern and authoritative administrative action enforcing uniform standards and introducing direct management of the health sector would run counter to the traditions of both institutional pluralism (Landau 1969), competition, and government by contract (see chapter 2). Nor must we forget that the dimension of competitive individualism was much in evidence when the first steps were taken to retrench the exorbitant national health bill, as demonstrated by the flourishing of health maintenance programmes sponsored by private employers.

The two central dimensions of American culture have both been at work in the long and slow war of attrition fought against the American Medical Association (Marmor 1983). The great esteem in which this powerful group had been held for so long started to vanish when the medical profession began to be perceived as possessing the quality and exhibiting the behaviour of a monopoly – certainly a bad word in the vocabulary of the sectarians, and not a particularly good one in that of the individualists either.

The counter-measures that were undertaken were not meant as a punishment meted out to an elite *qua* elite, but as a set of constraints and incentives capable of inducing that elite to correct its behaviour to the best of its ability and competence. Thus, the diagnostic-related groups can be seen as an injection of competition, as a way of breaking a monopoly more to the point than that which Friedman (1962) advocated by proposing a total deregulation in the 'production' of physicians.

Considerations of a similar nature can be developed to interpret other measures that are taken by many to imply a degradation, if not the demise, of clinical autonomy. I have in mind those governmental interventions that have introduced a variety of procedures centred on the principle of peer review: utilization review, professional standards review organizations, and peer review organizations. With such interventions the government has not enacted authoritative norms to be punctiliously applied by ritualistic bureaucrats; on the contrary, it has defined policy goals that the physicians themselves are asked to implement using to the best of their abilities their scientific knowledge and technical expertise.

This can hardly be described as heavy-handed treatment of professionalism. Neither could the methods adopted by governmental authorities in pursuing cost containment be called arbitrary and/or hierarchically characterized. The prolonged struggle between government and the doctors' guild can be depicted as possessing the nature of an open adversary relationship, if not formally, at least *de facto*. As a significant example, the federal bureaucracy relies on a faction of physicians to support the standards against which to measure medical practice (Anderson and Shields 1982).

Also, the federal bureaucracy has developed a considerable capacity for detail and methodological rigour, as demonstrated by such high-quality experimental work – fully utilized by the Washington agencies – as that produced by Yale University and by the New Jersey State Health Department (Marone and Dunham 1983). Finally, as Björkman puts it, 'HCFA has emerged as a well-insulated bureaucratic agency with a public service mission and a formidable set of skills' (chapter 2), which can be taken to mean that the government, rather than imposing bureaucratic edicts, has learned to speak the same language as its counterpart. It is one of those rare cases when a bureaucracy is guided by an experimental-empirical approach rather than by an unfortunately only too frequent goal-displacing deductivism.

**Conclusions: Organizational Rationality
and Medical Professionalism**

My concluding remarks stem from three premises that have been discussed in some detail in the foregoing sections and that can be succinctly stated as follows:

1 Nowadays, the delivery of medical services is a complex

collective endeavour which inevitably takes place in more or less formally structured organizational environments if it is adequately to perform its functions.

2 Mass access to modern health care occurs in a number of ways consistent with different cultural and institutional configurations of public intervention. This, in turn, has caused governments to tackle the problem of how to contain costs without degrading the level of health care.

3 Medical autonomy – in its conventional interpretation – almost everywhere is said to be endangered by the above-mentioned developments. Indeed, this conclusion would appear to be inescapable if we accept the notion that medical professionalism is a function of clinical autonomy *defined as individually independent practice.*

At this juncture, therefore, taking simultaneously into account these three propositions, the central questions are as follows. Is there an alternative interpretation of medical professionalism congruent with the organizational constraints of contemporary clinical practice? Which organizational format, among several possible alternatives, is more likely to provide operational conditions compatible with the deployment of medical professionalism?

To sum up the import of these questions in more specific language I suggest that the problem confronting us is that of determining which type of *organizational rationality* is more hospitable to the requisites of medical decisions and work processes. Distinguishing rationalities, in fact, relates directly to distinguishing decisions because, for different types of situations, we need organizational structures that permit the most 'rational' types of decisions (Freddi 1986: 167). Following Simon (1947, 1960), decisions formulated within organizational constraints are a function of both fact and value; that is, factual warrants are employed in establishing and justifying decisions. Therefore organizations can be classified according to the specific rationality which should inform their processes of decision and, accordingly, the appropriate structural configurations and procedures can be identified.

One such classification (Freddi 1986: 168) can be obtained by focusing simultaneously on the predispositions which give rise to organizational goals (the value dimension of decisions) as well as on the instrumentalities and process laws that qualify organizational means (the factual dimension of decisions). By and large bureaucratic and service organizations (health systems are certainly classified among the latter) tend to be characterized by goal consensus, by rather well-defined and unambiguous objectives. Where, on the contrary, these organizations tend to differ is in the degree to which they can rely on the adequacy of their instrumentalities.

The former can take it for granted that their means are adequate, up to their institutional task domains. The latter, on the contrary, have to do with task domains characterized by uncertain and problematic situations; these require constant adjustments and upgrading of the organizational means, of the knowledge necessary to run the organization, searching for effective and efficient performance.

In the first case we have organizational structures modelled after the classic Weberian bureaucracy. They are guided by codified norms; their modes of action aim to be reliable, predictable, and certain. In their thoroughly programmed contexts, to manage is the same as to control from a rigid hierarchical vantage point, to make sure that actions have been undertaken in accordance with previously and precisely defined parameters. In sum, these organizations are cast in the mould of legal rationality, conducive to synoptic, syllogistic, and deductive processes leading to authoritative decisions in an environment where goals are unambiguously defined and means fully adequate.

The picture is altogether different in the second case, that of service organizations concerned with goals that involve the employment of sophisticated technology and scientific procedures. By definition, in these organizations the participants charged with the pursuit of institutional goals – in our case the physicians – deal with uncertain and problematic situations. Dealing with such situations unavoidably entails a high probability of error. Since errors will occur inevitably, and cannot be prevented by introducing stringent, detailed, and authoritative bureaucratic rules, the problem then is not to make organizations error proof (an impossibility) but rather to make them error resistant.

In fact, the appearance of errors signals a structural inadequacy – that decision rules have not been up to scratch. If the organization is aware that errors are probable, and has been equipped with the appropriate monitors, then steps can be taken to find a correction. Constant corrections mean that an organization is continually modifying structure so as to reduce the probability of error (Landau 1973; Wildavsky 1972). The self-correcting organization is guided by a type of rationality which has very little to do with legal rationality. This experimental rationality involves incremental and pragmatic processes, leading to effective and efficient decisions, provided that the adequacy of organizational means constantly undergoes the empirical test.

My contention is that an organizational structure possessing the properties that have been just described is congruent with the requisites of medical professionalism. It is not individual decision-making that must be safeguarded – as the conventional notion of autonomy has it – so much as work processes that focus on exper-imental and empirical procedures competently controllable by peers. Hierarchical control is what must be avoided, not professional con-trol congruent with the training and socialization of all concerned organizational participants. Continuing in this vein, my reading of the several forms of public intervention recently evident in the US is that they do not debase professionalism. Quite the contrary: they create conditions leading to a controllable quality of mass health care.

Parenthetically, one might argue that in the same way that judges are granted independence not for their own gratification but to protect the citizenry from arbitrary and capricious actions, so the requisites of medical professionalism are inherently valid only as long as patients' care is the central objective. For example – as Harrison and Schulz point out in chapter 9 – the recourse to second opinions in difficult clinical cases is perceived as an infringement of medical autonomy. However, there is another side to this coin: second opinions introduce the beneficial principle of redundancy (Landau 1969), thus augmenting the probability of error avoidance.

In the words of an author who combines high-level clinical experience with a scholarly interest in the organizational aspects of medicine:

> A system of peer review for quality assessment pursues several different objectives. One is to identify and correct dangerous practices which might be involved in inadequate patient care. Another is the identifi-cation of procedures and practices which, while safe, may not be effec-tive in the treatment of particular illnesses and therefore unnecessarily costly. A third is to identify wasteful but useful practices which could be improved with both the saving of money and improvement in patient care. A fourth is to provide a system for medical personnel to use data from their own practices to constantly improve the effectiveness and efficiency of their own medical care by means of a system of monitoring to fit that person's own medical practice. Any or all of these goals and objectives might be included in a single effort to assess quality of care . . . PSROs have had a very major effect on the use of inappropriate and/or unnecessary injectible drugs . . . The effect on quality can be very significant. (Perkoff 1984: 84–5)

The introduction of peer review has not drastically changed American medical practice but, rather, has brought to their logical conclusion specific procedures established a long time ago, as in the case of monitoring of physicians in hospital accreditation systems. Nothing, or almost nothing, of this sort is to be seen in Europe, with the possible exception of some measures which are being introduced in Britain (see chapter 9). Thus the case considered by Döhler (chapter 8), whereby public organizational density is not detrimental to the conventional notion of clinical autonomy, seems well grounded. At this point, however, I would submit three observations:

1   One should like to know the effects of clinical autonomy (as individually independent practice) on the quality of health care, especially when there are rigid budgetary constraints determined in a general and abstract manner by some central governmental agency.
2   Nearly all European public health systems have adopted organizational structures that, in varying degrees, exhibit the traits of classic bureaucracies, such as centralization, distance between the decision-makers and work processes, and the like. Here, in connection with the notion of clinical autonomy, one is reminded of the latent properties of the 'bureaucratic phenomenon' so lucidly expounded by Crozier (1964), namely the protection of organizational participants from the anguish, anxiety, tensions, and conflict inherent in the face-to-face relationships typical of relevant controls exerted directly in the workplace. From this perspective, European physicians lead quieter and more serene lives than their American counterparts.
3   Finally, a bureaucratic, hierarchical approach to organizing health systems may very well spill over – with dysfunctional consequences for health care – in the work process itself, as a French study has pointed out (Kuty 1973; commented upon by Crozier 1986).

A final point should be made regarding the professional properties of health systems *qua* systems, by expanding and commenting on the arguments set forth by Hollingsworth in chapter 10. The US seems better equipped to meet the challenge of a mass access to costly and technologically sophisticated health care; this is thanks to the American tradition of institutional pluralism, which is very visible also in the modes of public intervention in the health sector (see chapter 2).

By and large, when European political systems have intervened, they have opted for centralized monopolistic bureaucracies that are, by their complexity alone, extremely susceptible to displacement of goals. They are not experimental, they do not learn easily and quickly, and their repertoire of responses is severely limited. This is what Hollingsworth discovered when studying the British case.

Its capacity for innovation and its adaptability to technological development is very low, whereas the opposite applies in the US.

The US, as we have seen, has a political tradition pluralist in character, hostile to monopoly and hierarchy and quite hospitable to the multi-organizational form. Formal coordinative devices are not thought to be very significant in establishing performance; preference goes to 'innovative spirit, flexible response capacities, error-correcting procedures, stable informalities, bargaining and redundancies' (Landau 1985). As we observe the first impacts of recent federal interventions in the health sector, we realize that some of these trends are already in evidence – provided we succeed in rejecting a first impression of inchoate dispersion.

2

Politicizing Medicine and Medicalizing Politics: Physician Power in the United States

James Warner Björkman

A Vantage Point on Control

Political control involves power, which is the ability to influence patterns of behaviour and to make others do (or not do) what they would rather not do (or do). A power relationship is inherently asymmetrical; if both parties to the relationship have equal power, neither can make the other change behaviour patterns. Different methods exist of holding others accountable for their actions, methods which can be classified non-exclusively as political, economic, bureaucratic, professional, and legal accountability (Björkman and Altenstetter 1979). In terms of resources for sanctions and decision rules, these mechanisms rely respectively on political norms (such as majority voting or civil obedience), bilateral exchange (such as money), hierarchical authority (such as rules), social status (such as self-policing), and the rule of law.

The members of any profession – or at least its preponderant majority – have 'some common ways of perceiving and structuring problems and of attacking and solving them; . . . are likely to share their views of the world and of the place of their profession in it; [and] . . . are likely also to share a common, and more or less unique, bundle of techniques, skills and knowledge, and vocabulary' (Mosher 1978: 147). These shared attributes are generated and sustained by self-recruitment, by educational training, and by socialization on the job within a given organization or series of organizations. Professional education is particularly important because the pressure of university academics has generated more and more theoretical and research-oriented knowledge as well as more and more fragmented specialities. It has been increasingly observed that such highly specialized university training does not provide much that is useful to effective practice; but corrective action takes place on the job as freshly minted apprentices unlearn and adapt their knowledge. Nonetheless, most professions continue to stress their links to specialized higher education and pressures continue to make educational requisites ever higher and more specialized. These links are still needed to justify a profession's claim to exclusivity, eliteness, autonomy, and self-governance.

Professionals who believe in the rectitude and relevance of their specialized knowledge, influence the course of governmental action and policy implementation individually as well as in concert with others. The principal (though not necessarily mutually exclusive) channels whereby they do so are:

1 Through the appointment or, more rarely, election of professionals to high office
2 Through effective control by individual professions of the significant managerial positions in administrative agencies
3 Through professionals who operate within agencies which they do not directly dominate
4 Through indirect pressures brought to bear on political executives and legislative bodies – that is by lobbying, professional associations, mobilized experts, the media, publication of research results, and so on
5 Through the network of professional ties (old boy, school, associational) across the boundaries of separate governmental organizations and agencies.

Drawing on a series of symposia in the *Public Administration Review*, Mosher (1978: 146) subjectively classified a dozen professions by the relative importance of these five channels of influence and concluded that, of these, 'the control of a specialized professional agency is the most frequent, and probably most important, channel of professional influence.'

Professionals, while very important for the implementation of complex policies, cannot be politically controlled the way democratic theory ideally sets up accountability systems. For example, majority voting does not and cannot direct expertise; it is too crude, too fickle, and sometimes quite wrong in terms of canons of received scientific opinion. Of course, majority voting can restrict professionals from practising altogether by banning their activities or even their existence; and majoritarian law can levy penalties and sanctions that set broad parameters of conscionable conduct by professionals. But expertise is not subject to validation (or disproof/ rejection/falsification) by majority voting.

Economic accountability would seem a more likely method to control professionals, at least if a balanced market for exchanges could exist. But given the specialized knowledge and expertise on which a profession is based, the relationship between providers and consumers is inherently unbalanced. With few exceptions, the exchange relationship is asymmetrical; and it tends toward monopoly control of passive recipients. This asymmetry is particularly acute (and increasingly evident) in the health sector where conditions of disease, illness and/or death elevate the provider to semi-divine status while simultaneously reducing the patients to a state of dependency. The claims of knowledge and expertise produce a self-fulfilling prophecy.

How much political control, then, do physicians wield in society? What changes, if any, have occurred in the autonomy and self-regulation of medical professionals? Are professionals in public service subject to any degree of political control? If so, how? If not, why not? These broad questions are addressed by reviewing aspects of the American case. Since the topic is so vast and since micro-behavioural measures (not to mention empirical data) are in short supply, this chapter will at best provide questionable answers to these perhaps unanswerable questions. But the challenge of understanding and accounting for the (changing) power of physicians is a welcome one – and every journey begins with one step and then another. First, I will provide a brief background of my own interest and perspectives on this topic. Secondly, I will briefly review the growth of the power of medicine in the United States and how reciprocally the politics of medicine inexorably entered the public arena. Thirdly, I will itemize some major legislative initiatives of the past twenty years that deal specifically with the power of physicians and their professional autonomy. Fourthly, I will explore three successive government efforts to monitor and control the practice of medicine. And fifthly, I will try to reach some conclusion on the two-way tendency not only to politicize medicine but also to medicalize politics.

Background and Contextual Perspective

To summarize, during the past decade I have conducted several different research projects on the politics of the health sector. The initial projects dealt with the impacts of intergovernmental relations on health care in the United States (Altenstetter and Björkman 1978) and with the political context of comparative health planning (Altenstetter and Björkman 1981). The former examined the effects (direct, indirect, and reciprocal) of changes in child health policies at federal and state levels over 40 years; and the latter examined problems of effectively implementing health planning programmes in Europe and the United States. A second undertaking has investigated who governs the health sector in Western industrialized states (Björkman 1985a). And a third project is examining how health resources are allocated in Third World countries (Björkman 1985b, 1986).

Since 1978 in particular, my field research has been on the degree to which comparative policies for representing interests and for decentralizing activities in health planning, financing, and operations affect modes of decision-making, the degree of accountability, and public acceptance of decisions. Behind this research lies an explanatory political model, which derives from an observation that the health sector has historically been a 'private government'. With few exceptions the provision of medical services has until recently been a private matter between supplier and consumer, between doctor and patient. Power over well-being or personal health status was exercised by an active agent with specialized knowledge over a passive recipient without such knowledge or expertise. The concept of self-care obviously lies outside this political framework, although one might argue that the very act of removing oneself from a dyadic relationship is itself a political act. The novel change in recent history has been the readiness of governments to enter the domain of hitherto private relationships in order to regulate the behaviour of both sets of actors (providers and patients). The political mandate of proactive governments is exercised through their administrative machinery. In the present era, government agencies take the form of bureaucracies with specialized roles based on the division of labour; these agencies, in turn, are hierarchically arranged and accountable both within the organization and sometimes externally to political leaders.

Consequently, there are four broad categories of relevant actors in the health sector of contemporary nation states:

1 The political leaders or politicians who represent – whether badly or adequately – the preferences and views of the 'people'
2 The administrators or bureaucrats who serve – whether badly or adequately – the political leadership
3 The professionals who, based on their expertise and training, provide the health care – usually medical services *per se*
4 The patients or clients who receive and/or consume these health services.

Since all flesh is mortal and subject to disability, decay and ultimately death, the fourth category subsumes the other three at some time or another in the life cycle. Hence the fourth category is also equivalent to the public who comprise the whole population. However, given the automatic constraints or liabilities of attentiveness (distraction) and size (disorganization), the fourth category is residual in the political model of the health sector (Krause 1977; Björkman and Silver 1978; Leichter 1979).

Given that all humans have health needs at one time or another in their lives, each of these broad categories of actors has specific roles (that is expectations as well as patterns of behaviour) attached to it. The politicians set the stage by choosing among alternatives (if any) in order to establish the goals for health care; they thereby legitimate the system of health services. Politicians also raise resources (financial, material, and human) and allocate them to the health sector – which is necessarily in competition with other sectors of government that seek these resources. The politicians can set the stage by inaction as well as by action, since they either acknowledge and reinforce the status quo or by default delegate the decision-making to other actors in the system. By their own actions in seeking help, members of the public can influence the pattern of health services; they can also raise some resources independently of the government (such as by voluntary labour or direct payment). Sometimes the government and the public are at loggerheads in that the former tries to change the latter's behaviour. For a variety of reasons, however, most of the public acquiesce in government decisions although they do not necessarily support them actively. Also, if the political leaders in government exceed the limits set by an acquiescent, tolerant people, then those leaders will be replaced. At least in the relatively democratic polities under consideration, these assumptions seem necessary and viable.

The roles of the bureaucrats are somewhat simpler, although they, too, can by default resemble those of the politicians. That is, while a bureaucracy is intended to be instrumental in carrying out the orders of the government (themselves based, however tenuously, on public mandates), the bureaucrats also can and often do pursue political roles. The study of implementation in the policy process has clearly suggested that even more political activity occurs within the bureaucracy and among administrators in relation to their peers and outside pressures (such as interest groups) than in the phase of policy formulation and legislative legitimation. Aspirations among bureaucrats and administrators to obtain recognition as professionals further complicate their roles in the health system.

The professionals who provide health (medical) services have critical roles in the whole health system. As long as health care remains invasive, based on specialized knowledge, and the product of dyadic relationships, the medical professionals will continue to influence the health sector. Some of the providers of health care are 'less professional' in the sense that they have less training and greater interchangeability; but all providers aspire to (if they are not already recognized as holding) professional status, and are the point of first contact for a patient in the health system. That is to say, whether curing or helping or even just caring, the health provider sits at the centre of the system. Try as they will, the politicians and the bureaucrats cannot replace the functions of the health professionals; and this centrality of function has been a source of power over all other actors. To be sure, various sanctions, penalties, incentives and rewards exist which can be used to channel and direct the behaviour of health providers. But – to belabour the obvious – one cannot provide personal health services without providers. Only the consumers or the patients themselves have the power to bypass the professionals by taking care of themselves; and such self-care, while possible through public education, widely disseminated information and shared knowledge, is really only supplemental to the direct invasive provision of health services.

Finally, the residual roles of the public are germane to the health system, but are more properly the province of medical sociology. General habits and attitudes toward health care do shape health behaviour – sometimes to the chagrin, lament and disgust of professional providers, bureaucrats and politicians. Hence, health care patterns must be understood and appreciated in psychosocial (cultural) context, whether one is looking at single case studies or in comparative terms. The one subset of patients or consumers of health care that merits special attention includes those who organize themselves into self-conscious, energetic groups. Each of the preceding categories – politicians, bureaucrats, and professionals – can also be internally divided into competing parties, associations, or interest groups; and such organization (usually) increases the power of these actors in the health system. Among the general public, however, the incidence of organized consumer groups is relatively rare and requires only occasional monitoring. Consequently, the patterns of performance in any health system can best and most efficaciously be described and predicted through the activities of relatively few active elite players operating within the contexts of culturally prescribed human behaviour.

Growth of the Power of Medicine in the United States

Control of medical standards and personnel

When the American Medical Association was founded in 1847, medical doctors (MDs) were only one of several types of medical practitioners using the designation 'doctor'. By modern standards medical practice at that time was primitive. Blood-letting and

amputation were common cures for a variety of ailments, while surgery was performed by barbers. As an association, the AMA sought
to improve the practice of medicine and to standardize the requirements of medical education. It sought to become a profession.

The first step in this process was a political effort to convince state
legislatures to license physicians. During the Jacksonian period of
populist democracy, many legal requirements for engaging in
professional practice had been abolished in favour of an egalitarian
'anyone-can-do-it' ethos (Gerstl and Jacobs 1975). From 1847 to
1900, medical examining boards were created in all the states. These
medical boards were, of course, manned by physicians.

With control over the practice of medicine established through
state regulation, the medical community pursued its educational
goals. Although the attempt to raise the educational standards of
medical schools was portrayed as an effort to protect the public's
health, historians have argued that the AMA's chief concern was
the number of physicians in practice and therefore in competition
(Shryock 1967). The AMA tied standards to the health issue by
arguing that many physicians were poorly educated and that the
nation only had resources to produce a limited number of quality
physicians. The public would be better off with fewer, better-
trained physicians.

Numbers are important, and their changes over time tell an
interesting story. In 1904 the United States had 164 medical schools,
many of which were proprietary. Because a proprietary school
increased its income by accepting more students, it had an incentive
to increase the size of its student body and to produce physicians as
quickly as possible. According to the AMA, this mill-like production of physicians led to low-quality practice, the very evil that
needed to be eradicated. In 1906 the AMA Council on Medical
Education examined the medical schools of the United States and
found that only 80 met the criteria of what a medical school should
be (Berlant 1975). Furthermore, 32 schools were completely
unacceptable (Kessel 1959). However, using such information to
restrict the supply of doctors was not feasible because the AMA
might be perceived as seeking economic gain for physicians at the
expense of the public.

To solve this credibility problem, the AMA persuaded the
Carnegie Foundation for the Advancement of Teaching to examine
medical schools. The Carnegie Foundation in turn hired Abraham
Flexner to do so, who was assisted in this effort by the AMA staff;
he also had access to the AMA's 1906 data. The conclusions of
Flexner's report in 1910 on medical education could have been
written by the AMA itself. Flexner concluded that too many doctors

diluted the quality of medical care. The public would be better served by fewer, better-trained doctors. Accordingly, many of the existing medical schools should be closed while those that remained open should restrict their admissions and adopt the uniform curriculum recommended by the AMA.

Armed with the Flexner Report as well as control over state medical examining boards, the American Medical Association proceeded to restrict entry to the medical profession (Kessel 1970). State medical boards required that a person graduate from a 'class A' medical school before he or she would be allowed to take the state medical exam. A class A medical school was one approved by the American Medical Association or the American Association of Medical Colleges. The schools on both lists were identical.

The AMA also asserted control over the internship process. Serving an internship with a hospital was a prerequisite to licensing. Hospitals – at least those controlled by physicians – required that a student graduate from a class A medical school in order to receive an internship. In combination these two factors restricted entry to the medical profession. A graduate of a non-accredited medical school would have difficulty finding an internship at an approved hospital. Without an internship, the student could not sit for the medical exam. Even with an internship at another hospital, the student might not be allowed to take the state exam because he or she failed to graduate from a class A medical school. The noose was complete.

The impact of these policies on medical education was striking. Faced with a system that refused to accept their graduates, proprietary medical schools closed. From 164 medical schools in 1904, the number dropped to 85 in 1920 and 76 in 1930. Schools with AMA approval restricted admissions dramatically. In 1905, 26,000 students were enrolled in medical schools, and 4,606 students graduated. By 1920 enrolments had been cut to 14,000 with 3,047 graduates – and yet, logically, the war in Europe should have increased rather than decreased demand for medical services. The impact of these cutbacks was so effective that the 1905 levels for students were not reached again until 1955. Not until the health care explosion of the 1960s that was inspired by federal government expenditures under Medicare and Medicaid did major increases in medical school enrolments occur.

The economic impacts of such restriction on entry to schools and, thereby, to the profession were dramatic. Physicians engaged in price discrimination by adjusting their fees to the income level of the patient. Some argued that such income-related fee adjustments allowed cross-subsidization wherein the better-off financed access to medical services for the poor. This was the classic posture of the brothers Mayo in their Rochester clinic – and the public approved. But as part of this desire to set prices arbitrarily without outside intervention, the medical community opposed innovations in health care delivery that were not based on individual fee-for-service arrangements. Prepaid health care plans were opposed by local medical societies, and doctors who participated in them were ostracized and denied hospital privileges (Kessel 1959: 33–41). Likewise, the AMA opposed free medical care for veterans in Veterans Administration hospitals as well as Medicare and Medicaid (Marmor 1973). The physicians engaged in a series of state-level battles with chiropractors, chiropodists, osteopaths, and midwives in order to restrict and even to eliminate these professions.

In effect, medicine became a closed society as far as consumers were concerned. It was not unknown, for example, that a doctor testifying for a patient in a malpractice suit would have future difficulties in using hospital facilities (Kessel 1970). Ironically, despite stated intentions to the contrary, all these restrictions did not result in health care indices superior to those of other, less restrictive nations. Although infant mortality rates and average life spans are certainly crude measures of health, those in the US fell far short of comparable indicators in many European countries. Possibly one reason why quality did not improve faster was the notorious 'grandfather clause'. By exempting current practitioners from new standards of training and performance, any impact of improvements on quality could only be incremental. Milton Friedman (1962) feels that AMA-imposed restrictions on entry have had such deleterious consequences that the nation would be better served if medicine were deregulated and the licensing of physicians were abandoned.

Medicine illustrates how a profession uses regulation that was proposed in the public interest for its own benefit. The situation in medicine was dramatically altered in the 1960s when the federal government became active in health policy. With the implementation of Medicare and Medicaid as well as various federal programmes to expand health care, health resources and health planning, control of the professions by the AMA was weakened. Health policy became too important to be left solely in the hands of doctors – although they still retain the preponderant influence (Fuchs 1974). Two indicators of federal impact on physicians' power over the supply of personnel are the increase in medical schools to 127 in number and the increase in medical students to over 66,000 today.

On the other hand, the shape of medical practice itself is

changing. As specialization has occurred, new organizations of specialist practitioners have been found which are increasingly in competition with the AMA itself. And when the state medical societies in the 1960s dropped the requirement that their members must also be members of the national association, the AMA experienced a dramatic decline in membership. Today less than half of America's certified physicians belong to the American Medical Association.

Control of medical fees and payment mechanisms
In 1900, before the advent of health insurance or federal regulation, doctors stood in direct relation to their patients as healers and benefactors. Neither private insurance companies nor government at any level had many regulations to guide medical practice. The demand for private health insurance became much greater after 1920 and intensified in the 1940s. It originated in the breakdown of the household economy as families increasingly came to depend on the labour of their chief wage earner for income. In addition, the ability of doctors and hospitals to provide efficacious medical treatment increased as the result of advances in medical technology and education. These two factors in turn caused the demand for more health insurance as the public sought to share risks.

Interestingly, from the vantage point of political analysis, the health insurer began to take on social and political roles as the importance of health insurance increased (Law 1974). From the viewpoint of physicians, all such private insurers represented an intrusion and a distinct break from tradition (Averyt et al. 1976). The 1940s and 1950s were periods of increasing constraints on the physicians, primarily through increased controls by the private insurers – among which Blue Cross and Blue Shield accounted for the greatest, most pervasive activity. The federal role was still very minor. Unlike the European nations, the United States took no action at this time to implement a national health insurance programme to subsidize voluntary funds or to make sickness insurance compulsory.

'In 1900, American government was highly decentralized, engaged in little direct regulation of the economy or social welfare, and had a small and unprofessional civil service' (Starr 1982: 240). At the national level, government had little to do with social welfare, and its health activities were minor. For example, Congress approved aid to mental hospitals in 1854, only to be vetoed by President Pierce; and it created the National Board of Health in 1879 but abolished it in 1883. Also, in 1798 hospitals for the merchant marine had been authorized and a number were subsequently built. Not until 1870, however, was the Marine Hospital Service formally organized as a national agency with a central headquarters. In stages in 1889, 1902, 1912, 1930 and 1944 Congress expanded the Marine Hospital Service and established the Commissioned Corps. But it gave them few functions and little authority; government health services were, in a word, minimal (Raffel 1980: 534–65).

Long before the provision of a national insurance programme to protect the elderly and indigent against the cost of medical care became an issue, the American public and Congress had engaged in a series of debates that addressed broader questions related to health insurance (Skidmore 1970). Serious public discussion of compulsory health insurance in the United States started around 1910, and continued in the 1930s and 1940s. When it was realized that compulsory health insurance would not pass if it were applied to everyone, a special tie-in with the aged emerged during the 1950s. By the end of that decade, health care for the aged had become a national political issue. It was tied to or embedded in the question of poverty, since many of the old were initially poor or became poor as they paid their expensive bills for increasingly needed medical care.

Immediately after his election, President Kennedy delivered to Congress the first presidential message ever devoted exclusively to the need for a health programme. In the message he strongly urged that hospital insurance for the aged be added to the social security system. After five years of intense congressional and public debate – and after the national trauma of a presidential assassination followed by an overwhelming electoral victory by the Democratic Party – the final Medicare legislation passed in 1965. National health insurance had come of age in America, even if for only a segment of the total population.

In establishing Medicare, Congress and the Johnson administration wanted to gain the cooperation of doctors and hospitals. To obtain this cooperation, two major decisions were taken. The first was to set up intermediaries to pay the hospitals. The advantage of using fiscal intermediaries was that it allowed for almost immediate implementation of the programme, and it eliminated the need for a separate government administrative bureaucracy.

The second decision involved the rules of payment for hospitals under Medicare. The legislation adopted the practice followed by Blue Cross of paying hospitals according to their costs. In basing reimbursement procedures on reasonable costs and charges, Congress also facilitated programme implementation. However, as time amply demonstrated, this reimbursement methodology contained no incentives for providers to control costs. In its desire to ensure access to care, Congress altogether ignored the problem of costs in the original legislation. Concern with access and quality of care soon gave way to legislative efforts to control costs, with a concomitant effect on the Medicare programme and its beneficiaries.

Legislative Initiatives and the Power of Physicians

It has been frequently argued that during the 1960s access was the most important concern, while during the 1970s and 1980s cost containment has become paramount. Federal legislation and, more importantly, federal regulations have mirrored these concerns. Federal trends from the early 1970s to the present clearly emphasize cost containment, although one must remember that prior to this time there had been very little federal regulation of health issues in the United States. Most federal health programmes had been voluntary and in fact patterned after the usual practice of federal–state cooperation in formula grants. The Hill-Burton Act of 1946 and its subsequent renewals provide the classic case (Raffel 1980: 588). Initially federal regulation was insignificant because the federal government itself had a limited role. Most power lay in the hands of the providers themselves. As the federal role increased, the decision to use the same system as private insurers and to use private insurance companies as intermediaries or fiscal carriers also tended to minimize government intervention. Consonant with its traditional political preference, the United States engaged in government by contract rather than direct government through state agencies. However, as government began to take the lead in cost containment efforts in the health sector, federal intervention increased. And the provision of medicine became increasingly politicized.

The federal government's involvement in health financing has grown enormously over the past twenty years as federal programmes have assumed responsibility for financing medical care to the elderly, the disabled, and the poor. Entitling these segments of the population to mainstream medical care has increased their use of services and improved their health. This also has increased the nation's total health bill. Likewise, public along with private insurance has fuelled rapid increases in medical prices and promoted increasing sophistication in medical care (Zubkoff 1976). As a result, the percentage of the gross national product (GNP) devoted to health care has grown each year to where it now represents 10.5 percent of the GNP.

Furthermore, health care cost inflation annually outpaced the average consumer price index for the past two decades. Although the rate has slowed in recent years, medical and hospital inflation still exceeds general inflation by more than half; in 1984 medical costs rose 6.1 percent (including a 7.4 percent rise in hospital room rates) while the consumer price index for all items rose only 4 percent (Pear 1985). Unsurprisingly, as early as 1969 the Secretary of the Department of Health, Education and Welfare (DHEW) called for measures to control health care cost inflation. Rising costs brought medical care under more critical scrutiny, and the federal government, as the major buyer of health services, began to intervene in new and unprecedented ways. The politicization of medicine continued.

As experts and politicians began to question whether more expensive services were worth the cost, the issue of cost containment supplanted improvements in access and quality on the federal policy agenda of the 1970s. During the first half of the decade Congress passed a great deal of complicated legislation, among which were temporary price controls as well as amendments to the Social Security and Public Health Service Acts. A brief chronology and discussion of these legislative enactments follow.

First, in August 1971 a general wage and price freeze brought a profound, but temporary, reduction in medical inflation. The wage and price freeze limited doctors' fees to annual increases of 2.5 percent and hospital charges to an increase of 6 percent. The general freeze was lifted in January 1973 but it was maintained for health care until 1975. Health care was singled out for special attention and additional regulation (Zubkoff 1976).

Secondly, in 1972 Congress passed a package of amendments to the Social Security Act that directly addressed the problem of rising health care costs and their effect on federal expenditures. Four major initiatives were involved that dealt, respectively, with hospital payments, capital formation, physician payments, and self-regulation of providers:

1   Some initial constraints were placed on federal payments to hospitals under the various programmes of the Social Security Act. Section 223 authorized the Secretary of HEW to establish methods for determining 'reasonable cost' of health services that takes into account 'various types or classes of institutions, agencies, and services'. An interim schedule of limits on hospital in-patient costs was published in the *Federal Register* in June 1974. Providers of health services immediately objected to these regulations as a method of imposing mandatory cost controls on

the nation's hospitals and as a means of meeting budgetary goals rather than screening for inefficient hospitals.

2   At the same time the federal government became involved in regulating health care capital formation and medical practice. Section 1122 of the 1972 amendments gave HEW power to deny full Medicare and Medicaid reimbursement to hospitals and nursing homes for any capital investment not approved by state planning agencies. For the first time, capital was something which the government monitored. As a consequence, health planning agencies achieved a negative or veto power over health care providers who received any federal funds under Social Security Act programmes – although proposals for capital expenditures under $100,000 were exempted.

3   The 1972 amendments also imposed ceilings on Medicare payments to physicians. The Secretary of HEW was authorized to develop an economic index for use in determining the amount of increase in physicians' fees that would be recognized for reimbursement purposes. Congress included this amendment in response to the astounding inflation in fees for physician services that had occurred since the passage of Medicare. Congress instructed HEW to create an index that would measure the increase in physicians' practice costs (such as the rental of office space or the wages of non-physician labour) and thereby permit an annual increase in income derived from Medicare payments that would be commensurate with the general rise in earnings in the United States. This medical economic index has been updated annually since its implementation, but the amount of increase in allowed charges has consistently fallen behind the consumer price index for all services and for physician services. That is to say, the actual increase in fees for physician services has always surpassed the percentage increase allowable under the medical economic index.

Furthermore, section 227 changed the basis for reimbursing teaching physicians in contrast to attending physicians. The original legislation (PL89–97) specified that all hospital services of physicians, except for residents and interns, would be reimbursed under part B of the Medicare programme. Hereafter teaching physicians would be reimbursed on a cost basis under part A (mandatory hospital insurance) rather than part B (optional physician insurance). The proposed regulations for implementing section 227 required a professional test (based on the physician–patient relationship) and a fiscal test (based on the payment profile of patients in the setting) in order to determine whether the billing allowed would be fee-for-service billing for attending physicians *or* cost-only billing for teaching physicians.

The opposition from organized medicine against section 227 of PL92–603 was so vehement that Congress again passed legislation in 1974 delaying implementation of section 227 until 1 January 1975. In the interim Congress authorized the National Academy of Sciences to conduct a study of appropriate and equitable methods of reimbursement for physician services under titles XVIII (Medicare) and XIX (Medicaid) of the Social Security Act. Although these studies were conducted, opposition to the limits imposed by section 227 continued. So-called 'final' regulations for this controversial measure were issued in the *Federal Register* on 11 March 1980, but never implemented. Instead the Omnibus Reconciliation Act of 1980 (PL96–449) repealed section 227 altogether.

4   Public Law 92–603 established professional standards review organizations (PSROs) in order to ensure that reimbursed services were medically necessary, provided in accordance with professional standards, and rendered at the appropriate level of institutional care. The country was thus blanketed with a network of PSROs. The law required that local groups of physicians be established to review the use of medical services and to control unnecessary utilization via either inappropriate admissions or unnecessarily long lengths of stay. Since local standards were used to determine the applicable criteria, differences in (for example) the average length of stay of more than two days between the east and west coasts were accepted. It is important to contrast this arrangement with the new prospective payment legislation (discussed more fully below) which, after an initial period of phase-in, is designed to have a single national standard. The regulatory process has moved from significant local autonomy where physicians established the standards to a more national direction with national standards.

The 1981 Omnibus Budget Reconciliation Act (PL97–35) required the Secretary of HHS (formerly HEW) to assess the relative performance of the PSROs. Numerous evaluations before and after the law indicated that the PSRO programme was only marginally effective. Consequently the 1982 Tax Equity and Fiscal Responsibility Act (TEFRA) repealed the existing PSRO programme and instead established the utilization and quality control peer review organization programme (UQCPRO). Since the acronym is unpronounceable, the name has been generally shortened to PRO. The new PROs are defined as either an entity composed of a substantial number of licensed physicians practising in an area, or an entity which has sufficient physicians available to conduct adequate peer review of medical services.

Thirdly, consonant with America's faith in economic liberalism, the discipline of the market-place was also invoked in order to control health costs. The Health Maintenance Organization (HMO) Act of 1973 and its 1976 revisions were aimed at stimulating competition among provider organizations. There has also been a trend toward deregulation elsewhere in the economy that has had indirect impacts. But interestingly, even business interests usually favourable to deregulation prefer to maintain some regulation (or even re-regulation) over the health sector (Pear 1985; *The Economist* 1985).

Finally, and very briefly, the early 1970s saw the passage of yet another law for systematic planning (see Altenstetter and Björkman 1981). The National Health Planning and Resources Development Act of 1974 (PL93–641 was actually signed into law by President Ford in 1975) established a tiered network of local and state health planning agencies which were guided by national directives promulgated by the Secretary of HEW. The Act absorbed, abolished and/ or reformulated several previous efforts at health planning – among them the Hospital Survey and Construction (Hill-Burton) Act of 1946, the Regional Medical Program of 1965, and the Comprehensive Health Planning Act of 1966 – and divided the country into health service areas. Each area was staffed by a health systems agency which produced local long-range health plans and annual implementation plans, all of which were reconciled by a state-wide health coordinating committee within federal guidelines. Although extended and amended several times, the 1974 planning act was chronically underfunded and it had little, if any, fiscal power. Its major leverage was to deny approval to capital expenditure projects financed by federal programmes under the Social Security Act. Nonetheless, PL93–641 was considered important because it monitored, albeit inadequately, the pluralistic American health sector, and because it was presumed to anticipate the structure for an 'inevitable' national health insurance. Wish fulfilment notwithstanding, national support for PL93–641 has now been terminated.

During the second half of the 1970s there was no major health legislation. Most of the political activity in health care financing involved implementing the Social Security Act amendments of 1972, such as tightening existing regulations to lower the maximum amount paid to hospitals under section 223. President Carter made hospital cost containment a high priority, but Congress repeatedly rejected versions of his proposal (Abernethy and Pearson 1979).

Many factors led to the demise of hospital cost containment legislation, including its complexity. Equally important, however, were the opposition of the hospital industry and the lack of significant taxpayer support. Because of the importance placed on the passage of hospital cost containment, no other significant legislative and regulatory initiatives in health care provision occurred during the Carter administration.

The federal government's inability to contain either public or general medical costs reinforced general reluctance to increase federal spending on health care. Certainly escalating health costs were a major impediment to the adoption of national health insurance during the 1970s. Neither national revenue controls nor national health insurance were enacted before President Carter left office, and the decade ended as it began – with health care absorbing a growing share of personal income and government budgets. The providers remained in control.

Nonetheless, throughout the 1970s prominent spokespersons for both political parties as well as a variety of analysts and commentators had advocated broader federal involvement in the control over health care financing. The differences among them concerned the methods used to control spending. Some advocated regulatory strategies; others sought the shock therapy of market discipline; still others pushed health education so that consumers and providers alike would practise self-restraint. The Reagan administration's objectives differed from earlier administrations in their emphasis on minimizing federal regulations, increasing responsibilities of the states and the private sector, and promoting competition and market-oriented reforms to promote efficiency.

The first major health legislation passed after President Reagan's election was the Omnibus Budget Reconciliation Act (OBRA) of 1981, which increased the responsibilities of the states and reduced federal regulation substantially. For example, states are now given much more latitude to design their own payment systems to pay providers in the Medicaid programme. Federal oversight and review procedures have been drastically reduced. OBRA was the first attempt of the Reagan administration to minimize federal regulation and to shift responsibility to the states.

Passage of the Tax Equity and Fiscal Responsibility Act of 1982 (TEFRA) initiated the next major reform of health regulations and the power of providers. One of TEFRA's most important changes was section 101, whose primary purpose was cost containment. Section 101 established new Medicare cost limits, effective October 1982, on total in-patient operating costs. The previous limits (from section 223, mentioned earlier) applied only to routine hospital costs and did not apply to ancillary services, which constitute about one-half of a hospital's bills. The TEFRA limits are established for each hospital under a case-mix index based on diagnostic-related groups (DRGs). In philosophical terms, TEFRA established the proposition that Medicare was buying a product from the hospital and that product is the treatment of patients with a certain medical condition (Marone and Dunham 1984).

Section 101 and other important provisions of the TEFRA legislation – such as elimination of the routine nursing differential, prohibitions of payment under Medicare for Hill-Burton free care, and recognition of the Secretary's authority to publish regulations eliminating the Medicare subsidy for medically unnecessary private rooms – all still maintained the principles of retrospective cost reimbursement. While TEFRA was an important first step in controlling the providers of health care, an additional step was required in order to obtain a full prospective payment system.

During 1982 the desire for increased competition and financial controls dominated thinking about federal regulations, and a series of subsequent health regulations were issued which had a significant impact on physicians and on the management of payments under Medicare. Two regulations stand out in particular. In order to implement section 108 of TEFRA, the *Federal Register* of 2 March 1983 published final regulations entitled 'Payment for Physician Services Furnished in Hospitals, Skilled Nursing Facilities, and Comprehensive Out-patient Rehabilitation Facilities'. The regulations distinguish in a very complicated way between physician services under parts A and B of Medicare and between teaching and non-teaching hospitals. In effect, however, by altering the computation of charges and determining the maximum allowable compensation, Medicare will not allow the non-teaching hospital to make a profit from physicians' services either.

The most dramatic and long-lasting change in reimbursement policy occurred in January 1984 with the publication of final regulations on Medicare payments to hospitals under TEFRA's diagnostic-related groups. The new DRG system has a transitional phase-in period of three years, but will produce profound changes in hospital behaviour. DRGs may also establish effective control over the fees of American physicians (see next section). One of the many studies mandated by Congress under prospective payment will explore the feasibility as well as the advisability of using a DRG-based approach to pay for physicians' in-hospital care of Medicare patients. While there are many fascinating questions in this study to be addressed by epidemiologists and accountants, the overriding political question is whether it is practical to link physician payment to DRGs. The Deficit Reduction Act of 1984 (PL98–369) required the Secretary of the Department of Health and Social Services to report to Congress by 1 July 1985 on the feasibility of DRG payments for physicians' services to hospital in-patients. Clearly the medicalizing of politics is proceeding apace.

On reflection, the history of Medicare and its impact on health care providers brings to light the evolutionary character of this particular government programme. The original design of Medicare, although never altered in its essentials, has been refined and modified to respond to the major health policy issues facing the nation at different times. The original concern with providing access to needed care produced a programme that covered the most costly forms of care (like hospital and skilled nursing services) and provided funds to support hospital and facility construction. The desire to protect other vulnerable members of American society such as the disabled and those afflicted with chronic kidney disease also resulted in the expansion of eligibility requirements for Medicare. However, the increasing cost of health care services and the proportion of those costs borne by the federal government have led to legislative and executive efforts to control costs through both new laws and supplemental regulations which limit reimbursement to providers and physicians. The current deficits in the federal budget have produced renewed efforts to achieve savings or reduce social expenditures by a combination of provisions that include increased cost sharing among beneficiaries, risk sharing on the part of providers, and cuts in the proportion of capital expenditures paid by the federal government.

Experiments in Controlling the Practice of Medicine

During the past twenty years the core political issue of the health care debate has been transformed from equity in access to containment of costs. Egalitarian principles were realized during the 1960s when public policy embraced the right to health care in the Medicare and Medicaid programmes. The demand for services generated by Medicare and Medicaid resulted in a gradual, but vast expansion of the nation's health care delivery system. The expansion in demand led, in turn, to soaring health care costs and growing fiscal concerns. By the mid 1970s national concerns had shifted from expanding access to health services to coping with the uncontrollable health care expenditures that resulted. By 1980, a seemingly irreversible political demand for health care budgetary restraints emerged in response to medical care inflation.

In traditional analysis, cost containment strategies can be subsumed under three categories: competition, public utility regulation, and centralized national health insurance (Marmor and Christenson 1982). In the past fifteen years Congress has attempted to control costs through a number of regulatory mechanisms associated with the first two categories. These regulatory efforts have met with limited success (Saltman and Young 1981). Policy-makers and health economists attribute the apparent failure of regulatory approaches to the fact that such mechanisms do not address the underlying problems associated with health care inflation, most specifically 'the unusual system of supply and demand' (Enthoven 1978). Unlike the pure market economy, where price is the controlling factor in decisions regarding the supply and demand for goods and services, consumers and providers in the medical market have been insulated against cost by third-party payment mechanisms and cost-based reimbursement. Moreover, whereas demand is controlled by consumers in the competitive market-place, physicians make the major decisions regarding consumers' need for goods and services. These perverse incentives operating in the medical market-place have led to 'market failure' in the health care industry.

Since the categories of competitive and regulatory solutions have not worked well (perhaps because they are more often than not mutually exclusive) and since a solution via centralized national health insurance has not been (and most probably will not be) tried in the United States, a fourth approach to controlling costs has emerged – that is, by limiting physician autonomy and the technical aspects of medical work. Congress has passed laws and authorized regulations that address the physician's central role in ordering medical services. As will be argued, state intervention has followed an increasingly intrusive path into the physician's once-private world of technical autonomy. The drive to control physician autonomy highlights the political nature of autonomy itself. Physicians control approximately 70 percent of health care resources by virtue of their legal monopoly over medical care (Nobrega and Krishnan 1983). Controlling the major group of controllers of health care resources is a public policy response to the cost containment imperative; limiting technical autonomy is the method.

Autonomy: the political bedrock of professional control
Until recently, physicians have enjoyed the privileges of professional autonomy on a comprehensive scale, including: control over methods of payment; control over the social organization of their work; and exclusive control over the content of their work, or technical autonomy. Four more privileges can be derived from technical autonomy: freedom from competition from non-physician

personnel; freedom to self-regulate; freedom to regulate the work of other related occupations, such as respiratory therapists; and freedom to regulate patients (Freidson 1975).

Based on the classical attributes of the definition of a profession – that is, special knowledge and a public service ethic – an assumption is made that the physician should act as an agent for the patient in ordering care and should be the final arbiter of medical work. This forms the ideological foundation of health services. However, these claims must bear a political endorsement through a government grant of autonomy before they can be translated into professional power and control over resources. Before the Civil War, for example, medicine's claim to the classical attributes was rejected by popular opinion, alternative practitioners and politicians alike (Gerstl and Jacobs 1975). Yet by the late nineteenth and early twentieth centuries, faith in medicine's special expertise had replaced this distrust; the change was signified by state licensure laws and medical education reforms (Starr 1982).

The point is that in order to secure autonomy, the medical profession had to enter the political arena and act as an interest group seeking to influence public policy to its own advantage. Much of the medical profession's power is based on the legally supported monopoly of practice which operates through a state government system of licensing, and that bears the privilege of exclusive patient management. Physicians have had an exclusive right to offer medical services and control access to the resources necessary to managing medical problems related to those services.

In order for medicine to maintain autonomy, physicians must continually re-enter the political arena to enlist the support of political decision-makers in maintaining their pre-eminence. Claims to special knowledge and a public-devoted ethic can be viewed as resources which, used initially to convince decision-makers that autonomy should be granted, again are used to buttress claims that it ought to be maintained. The role of the state is to maintain non-interventionist policies relative to health care services programmes. In a pluralistic political system, policy is a result of bargains struck among vested interests, with no one interest consistently dominating the decision-making (Feingold 1977). Physicians' interests have traditionally been recognized in the policy-making process.

However, to the degree that medicine is dependent on governmental units for its professional power, its autonomy is vulnerable to manipulation. The expansion of patient rights through the courts, which alter the doctor–patient relationship, is illustrative (Starr 1982: 388–91). The current Medicare restrictions on fee increases is another. In sum, it is not the medical profession that has sovereignty; rather it is the state that has sovereignty 'and grants it conditionally' (Freidson 1975: 24). Autonomy is the political core of the medical profession, and it can only be understood 'as the outcome of a political struggle to control key resources', including the autonomy itself (Björkman 1982: 415).

The issue of physician power and medical autonomy is always complicated because doctors practise in two distinct, if overlapping, arenas: the self-standing clinic (whether solo or group practice) and the hospital. Since much of the health money is channelled through hospitals, their internal power structure needs to be understood. Drawing on Crozier's model of organizational behaviour being determined by a conflictive power equilibrium, the hospital as a decision-making organization contains six major occupational groups: physicians, administrators, nurses, medical technicians, clerical personnel, and service personnel (Saltman and Young 1981). Each group has a stable but flexible group strategy designed to maximize its authority over decisions which affect that group. Each group attempts to increase its latitude within the hospital by maximizing other groups' uncertainty that it will perform its function as expected; but no group pushes its interest to the point of threatening organizational survival.

The primary decision-making struggle exists between physicians and administrators, a contest which effectively orders all other intergroup relations within the hospital. For example, physicians order relations through issuing medical orders, while administrators order relations by managing resources through a hierarchical chain of command. Physicians, however, are not a part of the hierarchical chain of command because they are paid by sources external to the hospital. As the folk formula puts it: 'Only doctors have patients; hospitals have only doctors.' The power struggle which emerges from this structural relationship is discussed below.

By virtue of their control over the major sources of unpredictability within the hospital's production process, physicians are perceived to be at the apex of power. Physicians are able to carve out their zone of autonomy through exclusive control over patient care: admissions, diagnosis, orders for tests and procedures, decisions on levels of care, and discharge. They therefore control three of the hospital's critical cost and revenue generating variables: admissions, clinical resource consumption, and length of stay. These are the central sources of unpredictability in the service production function. Besides the short-term impact on hospital production and finances, physicians exercise control over most capital costs, especially new services and technology. In terms of the financial survival of the hospital, physician behaviour is *the* critical variable.

The key decision-making struggle between physicians and hospital administrators pivots around the control of the variables that comprise the central source of unpredictability in the production function. These two major actors pursue different interests and are unequal in resources as they vie for control over the decision-making processes. The power equilibrium between the two changes only as the resources of one or both are altered.

The foundation of the physicians' crucial role in the hospital is their monopoly over technical expertise which effectively frees them from supervision by hospital management. By operating within a black box filled with the special knowledge that governs the medical decision-making process, to which only they are privy, physicians are able to 'maximize the uncertainty that they will perform their function as anticipated' (Saltman and Young 1981: 408).

In order for hospital administrators to strengthen their control over the hospital decision-making process, they must have access to the special knowledge comprising medical expertise. The same may be said of any would-be external regulator. With access to knowledge, norms could be developed by which physician performance could be measured, and management tools could be developed by which the degree of unpredictability in the production of hospital services could be decreased. One other requirement would have to be fulfilled before administrators could develop and apply these management tools – namely the political endorsement or stimulation of such activities. During the past two decades there have been three successive attempts in the United States to monitor medical practice and reduce physician autonomy.

Utilization review
Medicare was the culmination of a 35-year ideological polarized battle over national health insurance in the United States. The Democratic landslide of 1964 enabled the 89th Congress to pass that legislation, and both Congress and the Johnson administration were eager for the programme to be implemented quickly and successfully. To ensure the cooperation of physicians and hospitals who would provide medical services to the beneficiaries, Congress essentially grafted the Medicare programme on to the existing health care delivery system. Congress declared its intention of non-interference with the health care system in section 1801 of the law, entitled 'Prohibition against any Interference'. This so-called 'AMA clause' prohibited the federal government from exercising 'any supervision or control over the manner in which medical care services were provided . . . or . . . over the administration or

operation of any . . . institution, agency, or person' providing health services (Thompson 1981: 159).

This non-interference contract between the federal government and providers was backed up by a number of attractive incentives. The primary incentive was that payment rules were to conform to principles of payment being used by third-party payers, particularly Blue Cross and those condoned by the American Hospital Association (Feder 1977: 1). This amounted to reimbursement for 'reasonable costs' through hospital-nominated fiscal intermediaries. Programmatic responsibility was given to the Social Security Administration (SSA), which was the bureaucratic base of several Medicare strategists; and the majority of hospitals chose Blue Cross – their own creation and long-standing ally – to act as buffer between the hospitals and the well-disposed federal agency. Similarly, physicians were to be paid according to their 'usual, customary, and reasonable' fee through an intermediary, the majority of which turned out to be Blue Shield (Starr 1982: 375).

Both physicians and hospitals stood to benefit enormously from the increased earnings and guaranteed revenues to which few requirements were attached. Payments for care that once fell under the heading of non-reimbursed charity care were now ensured through a fiscally irresistible programme provided by the federal government. 'As a result, the administration of Medicare was lodged in the private insurance systems originally established to suit provider interests. And the federal government surrendered direct control of the program and its costs' (Starr 1982: 375). Yet as Congress and the administration had wished, the Medicare programme was launched quickly and successfully.

Despite the non-interference contract of the AMA clause, however, two requirements were built into Public Law 89–97. One concerned certifying hospitals which had to meet minimal quality standards; the other was utilization review (UR). The purpose of the UR programme was to ensure that physicians engaged in cost-effective treatment practices so that hospital resources would be used efficiently. Since physicians control approximately 70 percent of medical care resources via their exclusive control over patient management, it was clear to Representative Wilbur Mills – the powerful chairman of the House Ways and Means Committee – that controlling medical care costs required influencing physician behaviour (Anderson and Shields 1982: 26). Utilization review was the lever supplied.

The Medicare law mandated two types of review: general reviews of practice patterns in order to assure quality, and specific reviews of long stays in order to monitor the use of resources. As expected, organized medicine opposed utilization review from its inception on the grounds that it transgressed professional boundaries of autonomous control of medicine, specifically technical autonomy and self-regulation. After the law was passed, the AMA supported only reviews to assure quality because it regarded quality assurance as an educational activity. But the AMA remained unalterably opposed to utilization review of resources which it considered an illegitimate policy activity by the government (Feder 1977: 34–5).

Meanwhile, the Social Security Administration had no precedent from which to derive guidance in setting up such a review system. Previous quality review activities within the medical community were limited in number and in scope, and almost none existed before Medicare whose activities were directed toward efficient use of hospital resources (Covell 1980). Traditionally cost had not entered the physician's clinical decision-making process. Hence, there were not only no precedents but also no standards by which to measure inappropriate resource use.

However, the SSA had a third option for meeting the legal requirement of utilization review: the monitoring function could be delegated to state health agencies and/or fiscal intermediaries. The AMA, the AHA and Blue Cross strongly opposed federal government involvement via state agencies. It was argued that if state oversight was chosen, Medicare officials would evaluate utilization and their disallowances would threaten reimbursement. By contrast, reliance on fiscal intermediaries would tie oversight to the payment process itself. While the latter was in effect devoid of an enforcement mechanism, the role of Blue Cross would expand if fiscal intermediaries were used – as would their revenue (Ensign 1978: 188–91).

However, the primary objective of the Social Security Administration was to implement Medicare; and implementation required support from the providers. Furthermore, there were neither precedents for how to develop the programme nor criteria by which to measure medical care utilization. From past experience with the social security trust funds, SSA was a payment processing agency; the monitoring of physicians was clearly out of its area of expertise. Consequently the SSA took the path of least resistance offered through a balancing strategy to achieve its objectives.

The balancing strategy resulted in a review system developed and controlled by committees composed of physicians at the hospital level. State agencies were authorized to conduct procedural reviews of utilization review committee activities, but primary responsibility for substantive evaluation was given to the fiscal intermediaries. The claims review process of these intermediaries did not include a

substantive review of practice patterns, the lack of which incapaci-
tated any potential enforcement of the law.

All of this was consonant with the non-interference clause of
the Medicare Law. Presumably utilization review was included
in PL89–97 because of Congressional concern about potential
increases in cost. However, enforcement of this provision of the law
would have required that SSA challenge the medical community
and thereby undermine the overriding objective: implementation of
a federal health insurance programme in the United States. Political
costs would have greatly outweighed political benefits. By delegating
programme responsibility to fiscal intermediaries and independent
utilization review committees, the Social Security Administration
avoided such a direct challenge of physician power. Indeed, a
passing remark by Representative Mills clarifies the intent of
utilization review and conveys the spirit of the entire Medicare Act:

> Shortly after the passage of the Medicare Act, one of the architects of
> that legislation was asked the following question: In the preamble to the
> Medicare Act there is a statement that the Act will in no way interfere
> with the private practice of medicine, yet in a few paragraphs later there
> is mandated that each hospital set up utilization review committees to
> monitor length of stay. 'Is this not interfering with the private practice of
> medicine?' Rep. Mills smiled and leaned back in his chair: 'Oh, no, that
> provision in the law is simply to make doctors talk to each other'.
> (Anderson and Shields 1982: 126)

During these first years of the Medicare programme, physicians and
hospital administrators shared a coincidence of economic interests
under cost-based reimbursement operations. Physicians earned
more for providing services in the hospital than in an out-patient
setting. Additionally, the greater the volume of services and the
more complex the individual procedures, the greater the compensation earned. Maximizing the key clinical variables – that is,
admissions, diagnosis, levels of care, tests and procedures, and
length of stay – could be translated into maximum earnings. Simultaneously, maximizing physician income also meant maximizing
hospital revenues. The prescribed reliance on fiscal intermediaries
for oversight left control over utilization review activities within the
hospital itself; and the results were as expected.

During the era of utilization review, physicians generally did not
criticize each other, especially given the conditions of clinical
uncertainty under which they operate (Blumstein 1976: 264). The
overlay of Medicare financing incentives did not enhance the
attractiveness of this proposition. Yet there were no agreed
standards governing the clinical variables of patient care by which
criticisms of overutilization could be lodged. If the Social Security

Administration had wanted to intensify utilization review activities – which it did not – lack of knowledge would have provided a formidable constraint, if not indeed one that would have made this venture impossible.

As Medicare became an 'uncontrollable' budget expense, policy-makers had to confront choices about utilization and payment schedules more seriously than they had in 1965. But government officials were not alone in their desire to control the health care sector. The 1970s were characterized by increasingly enlightened consumers who demanded accountability from a health care system perceived to be inequitable, inefficient, and of questionable utility (Krizay and Wilson 1974). Employers paying high health premiums, as well as the commercial insurance industry concerned with its own competitive edge against Blue Cross, also began to favour compre-hensive reform (Starr 1982: 383–8). Furthermore, health services research began to report that physicians scheduled unnecessary surgery and that hospitalization rates varied sharply across regions. It became increasingly clear that the role of the physician was central to any public consideration of limiting medical expenditures. And a political coalition was coalescing to attempt greater control over the practice patterns of physicians.

Professional standards review organizations
Proposals for review of medical care began to surface in the late 1960s from various quarters, including federal agencies and the AMA itself. But the major impetus for change emerged primarily from Senator Wallace Bennett of Utah, the ranking Republican member of the Senate Finance Committee (Feder 1977: 43–5). Bennett's objective was to control medical services by influencing medical practice, and he proposed that the review process be conducted by local physician groups accountable to a federal agency rather than by the fiscal intermediaries. The AMA objected to provisions of his proposal involving government ownership of records, mandatory advance approval for elective surgery, and national norms for health care. But with several modifications, Congress enacted the professional standards review organization (PSRO) programme in the Social Security Act amendments of 1972.

The modifications secured by the AMA were critical to physicians maintaining control over the technical aspects of their work. The status of pre-admission certification for elective surgery was changed from mandatory to voluntary. The final legislation restricted PSRO responsibilities to institutional service, thereby constraining the scope of review activities. Furthermore, only physicians could participate in programme decisions; and the government would not own the data. Altogether medicine managed to retain control over the PSRO programme.

Nonetheless, members of the medical community expressed indignant outrage both before and after the PSRO legislation was passed. They protested that the law would ultimately force physicians to practise medicine by averages; that the programme's primary objective was cost control rather than quality assurance; that the programme put the doctor–patient relationship and its confidentiality into jeopardy; and that the programme would cost more than it would save (Lebish 1982: 992).

The legislation itself clearly contained conflicting goals of quality assurance and cost containment, but the *Congressional Record* records that Senators Bennett and Russell Long advocated an educational emphasis for PSROs. This attitude evolved into the articulation of quality of care as the primary objective of the new law. Like administrators of the utilization review programme, officials of the Office of Professional Standards Review (the federal agency implementing PSROs) adopted the posture that Congress had advocated. Their pliancy dovetailed well with the AMA position that, under conditions of conflict between cost and quality issues, maintenance of quality was to be the primary objective of peer review (Blumstein 1976: 248–9). Also the AMA insisted on local decision-making about norms of medical care rather than the imposition of national or even regional standards.

Implementation of the PSRO programme was marked by considerable delay. Programme administrators, hospital review committees and PSROs themselves were uncertain about how to proceed. Lack of a model system for monitoring medical care accounted for the delay as much as resistance by the physicians. As it turned out, neither of the two major methodological options for setting standards – empirical or statistical – produced reliable indicators. And the computerized utilization review system developed by OPSR required technology that many hospitals did not own at the time (Thompson 1981: 144–5).

Consequently, despite claims (or fears) to the contrary, PSROs did not impose negative sanctions on physicians. The educational slant of the programme, the conceptual quagmire of setting standards, the technicalities written into the law by Congress, and the political constraints involved in peer disapproval, all contributed to the de-emphasis on sanctions. Furthermore, federal administrative activities were confined to procedural matters rather than substantive concerns; and federal administrators had little control over the programme.

Early in the Carter administration the PSRO programme was

found to be cost ineffective because its emphasis on quality assurance tended to inflate services rather than constrain them. In response to this criticism, the programme was relocated in the Health Care Finance Administration (HCFA) in 1978. Despite intensified administrative efforts to induce PSROs to conduct vigilant reviews or 'be defunded and replaced', relocation had little effect on changing the programme emphasis from quality to cost control (Lebish 1982: 992). A Congressional Budget Office report in 1979 condemned the programme as a cost containment failure; and it was slated to be phased out by 1981 under President Reagan's proposed economic recovery Act.

In the cases of utilization review and PSROs, programme outcomes are consistent with historic government action in the health system. State authority was simply delegated to the medical community. Physicians were responsible for developing, implementing and overseeing the programmes; and the federal government, in the main, served merely to endorse their activities. Most of this delegation (or abdication, as some would have it) of authority was not inconsistent with Senator Bennett's vision of the PSRO programme. The point of the legislation was to place peer review under physician control in order 'to enhance their [physicians'] stature as honorable men in an honorable vocation' and to protect the public interest in cost containment and quality assurance 'while at the same time, leaving the actual control of medical practice in the hands of those best qualified – America's physicians' (quoted in Blumstein 1976: 248). Yet Bennett and others also viewed the PSRO programme as the last opportunity for the medical community to take control of the quality *and* costs of medical care before someone else assumed responsibility for these objectives.

Like utilization review previously, the PSRO programme was absorbed by the power structure of hospitals. The resistance to the programme by both physicians and administrators derives from their desire to maintain and increase their zones of autonomy, and from each group trying to maximize its control over decisions which affect it. Any externally imposed review system injects an element of uncertainty into the hospital revenue maximizing scheme, and reduces the administrators' already limited control over the major variables of the production process. Hence the American Hospital Association demanded that PSRO review responsibilities be delegated to the hospital committees, just as it had resisted oversight in the utilization review programme.

Resistance by physicians to the programme emerged from the limits to technical autonomy imposed by an external review system. PSRO utilization activities concentrated on admissions and lengths of stay; PSROs used regional norms and standards adjusted to local conditions to determine the appropriateness of the clinician's judgement (Goran 1979). Resistance to the programme revolved around the questions of who is clinically correct: the individual practitioner, the local group, the regional aggregate, or the national average. Opposition to PSROs was thus in part a manifestation of professional resentment to external supervision of a process that had traditionally been insulated from outside review.

A more principled objection concerned the underdeveloped techniques for measuring efficiency in medical care. There simply were no operational definitions for over- and underutilization of services. The norms were based on averages which imply a judgement that the average case is of adequate quality (Anderson and Shields 1982: 125–53). Both the PSRO officials and the federal administrators were sensitive to this problem, as were the local physicians to whom the review system was applied. Since individual physicians are (or were) the only owners of medical knowledge and judgement, they have a duty as final arbiters of medical care to employ those faculties when confronted with an individual case.

Little information has been collected on changes in physician behaviour as a result of the PSRO programme; and the validity of those evaluations conducted are questionable (Rosen 1978: 48–63). Each hospital and each physician has a profile of statistical information that the PSRO gathered, but this information is confidential. Once the data are aggregated to the point where individual hospitals and physicians are not recognizable, they can be published. But aggregate shifts on the macro level do not permit analysis for change on the micro level. Hence it has not been possible to assess the programme's impact on physician practice patterns.

Several things, however, are known for certain to have changed. First, technical autonomy was indeed decreased under PSROs. Clinical decisions of individual physicians were reviewed by physician groups, including Medicare-related (after the fact) admissions, level of care determinations, and lengths of stay for outliers. Previously physicians had enjoyed the professional prerogatives of individual self-regulation within formal and informal constraints. Formal constraints included legal and professionally promulgated ethical rules; informal constraints included the exclusion of 'bad physicians' from peer referral. PSRO activities transgressed all these boundaries.

Secondly, PSRO brought about massive physician participation in peer review activities. For the first time physicians on a grand scale reflected on their practice patterns in terms of cost versus benefits to the patient. Quality and utilization review techniques evolved from a point of little precedent to computerized profile analysis and problem-oriented quality review. In sum, the PSRO programme accomplished the hope that Representative Wilbur Mills had for its utilization review predecessor: it got physicians to talk to each other.

Medicalizing politics: PROs and DRGs

During the 1970s and into the 1980s medical care inflation continued at double-digit rates. These heightened demands for government intervention to control health care costs, which became a prime focus of attention in the political arena. Employers, the insurance industry, the health care critics, all disillusioned with previous regulatory efforts characterized by provider dominance and regulatory ineffectiveness, demanded a more potent cost containment solution. If costs were to be controlled, government was expected to find the way.

Against the background of demands, Congress was confronted simultaneously by an exorbitant health care bill and an ever-widening gap between federal expenditures and revenues. Medical care inflation was outpacing inflation rates in the rest of the economy, and doing so against what appeared to be a shrinking economic context. One of the most visible aspects of high inflation was the greater than average inflation in the hospital sector. The cost-based reimbursement system was perceived as supplying perverse incentives which fuelled the inflationary trend. By the late 1970s pro-competitive theories of health care economics were becoming popular (Enthoven 1978). Furthermore, the Medicare trust fund was being depleted. The political summation of these various factors led Congress to seek a solution in the form of prospective payment limits.

The solution was the prospective payments system (PPS) based on diagnostic-related groups (DRGs) plus the peer review organization provisions of TEFRA. Under PPS, hospitals are paid according to a prospectively determined fixed price per discharge for 467 different categories of illness. PPS is based on the theory that efficient hospitals whose costs per case are less than the standardized government payment will be rewarded; inefficient hospitals whose costs are more than the fixed price will be penalized. This pricing mechanism of 467 diagnostic-related groups was phased in over a period of three years, during which time the payment amount consisted of a blend of national, regional and hospital-specific rates. Between fiscal years 1984 and 1987, the basis for payments was transformed from primarily hospital-specific local rates to entirely national rates through the increasing assimilation and reconciliation of regional norms. All prices were based on statistical norms developed from Medicare billing statements (Hunt 1983).

The 1982 Tax Equity and Fiscal Responsibility Act (TEFRA) created a mechanism for overseeing the application of DRGs to medical practice. The utilization and quality control peer review organizations (PROs for short) are organizations of or sponsored by private physicians that contract with the Health Care Finance Administration (HCFA) in order to conduct quality assurance and utilization review activities. Most PROs are a combination of state medical societies and former PSRO groups which merged into a single state-wide organization (Wallace 1984). PROs are based on the same theory as the now-defunct PSRO programme. If a rational basis can be found for judging the quality and quantity of medical services, then a national basis can be found for justifying the cost of those services (Anderson and Shields 1982: 127). By implication, this rational basis could also serve to justify *not* providing services deemed inessential; therefore it could serve as a justification for withholding payments and reducing costs.

As conditions of their two-year federal contracts, each PRO is required to (1) review the reasonableness, necessity and appropriateness of hospital admissions; (2) review the completeness, adequacy and quality of care provided; (3) validate the diagnosis and procedural information that determines reimbursement; and (4) review the necessity and appropriateness of care for outliers for which payment is sought. Indeed, against a list of predetermined criteria, the physician must receive PRO approval for admission of patients or the hospital may not be paid for services rendered. These requirements are operationalized through PRO procedures designed to review and control, under specified conditions, all of the variables which together comprise medical care management – that is, admissions, diagnosis, tests and procedures, levels of care, and length of stay. Spokesmen for organized medicine argue that these criteria and requirements assume overutilization with its attendant ill effects on cost and health alike; and they argue that the objectives are based on standards and norms for which no professional consensus exists (Boulanger 1984).

The PRO can apply penalties or negative sanctions in a variety of ways if physicians fail to follow the bureaucratically prescribed path of process and/or adherence to standardized norms. For example, physicians may be disqualified from participation in Medicare – and last summer the Wisconsin PRO made an example of at least two physicians (*WiPRO Reviewer* 1984). However, it is the hospital (and some patients) which usually will be penalized for what HCFA considers to be service errors, through payment disallowances for resulting hospital costs that are greater than DRG payment.

The most outstanding aspect of the DRG programme is the transfer of power by Congress from physician and hospital providers to the federal bureaucracy. Like utilization review and the professional standards review organizations, the DRG solution emerged from within the federal government; but this time it was the federal bureaucracy, and not Congress, which produced the solution. In 1982 Congress had ordered the Secretary of Health and Human Services to develop a prospective payment system for Medicare; and the Secretary·responded with DRGs taken from the New Jersey experiment in which HCFA had been the least obvious but one of the most influential actors (Marone and Dunham 1983).

Diagnostic-related groups encapsulated a fairly attractive political package to policy-makers who had moved beyond the cost crisis rhetoric to the issue resolution stage. First, the DRG mechanism fitted the description of the Congressional mandate; it was prospective. Secondly, it appeared as a viable tool by which the federal government could control Medicare costs. Thirdly, it would not appear to equity-conscious consumer groups – particularly the aged – as a direct cut in access. Congress could control costs by capping 467 different treatment categories instead of limiting total costs and thus having to deal publicly with the trade-off between access and cost.

Finally, it was a solution that was available for an enormously complex public problem. Legislators rarely have the incentives, time or expertise to master the intractable problems plaguing the health sector. Furthermore, despite ten years of PSROs as well as extensive committee hearings on Medicare payments, during which Congress repeatedly told the AMA and other groups in organized medicine to develop a solution, the medical community had produced no cost containment strategies whatsoever. The DRG solution emerged in a kind of policy vacuum, and Congress turned to its traditional source of expertise and advice: the bureaucracy.

Hearings before the Subcommittee on Health of the Senate Finance Committee on 2 February 1983 reveal how the positions of the AMA and the Congress were juxtaposed. Based on its traditional opposition to rationing necessary medical care for cost containment purposes, the AMA stoutly opposed DRGs; it argued that while the method may appear politically expedient, DRGs were as yet unproved in their effect on medical care. Organized medicine recommended a period of experimentation and demonstration projects before DRGs were implemented. AMA spokesmen also recommended that Congress postpone action until the AMA had finished a research project currently under way, at which time Congress could then consider a proposal developed by those with special knowledge. Senator Robert Dole (Republican from Kansas and subsequently Senate Majority Leader) responded:

> Our problem is that Medicare is going to sink one of these days if everybody comes up here and tells us not to do anything this year, do it next year, or don't do it at all. If we think Social Security is in trouble, we ought to look at Medicare trust funds in the next 4 or 5 years. We have a very heavy responsibility on this committee to try to somehow get a handle on health care costs. They are about to eat us up. And we would hope that those who are directly involved would do more than suggest we delay it for another year. We can't delay it for many more years. We won't be around – Medicare won't be around.

Unquestionably Congressional interest in doing something about cost control outweighed any concern for the interests of the medical profession. The AMA 'party line' had lost its erstwhile persuasive appeal.

Somewhat in contrast, the official stand of the American Hospital Association was favourable to DRGs, but this position must be seen in the light of limited policy choices, a divided industry, and credibility issues. DRGs turned out to be the least coercive, and therefore the most desirable, alternative that HCFA had considered during 1982 (Marone and Dunham 1983). Furthermore, competition in the hospital sector stimulated during the past few years was already having a divisive effect on a once-united industry. Perhaps the most important and least obvious reason for the official AHA stance is credibility. Hospitals had received sustained and severe criticism in the press for their unreasonable rates. Hospital beds and services were more expensive than accommodations at luxury hotels. The usual industry response to the public and Congress was that hospitals had no incentive to keep costs down. 'Here's one,' said the Senate Finance Committee with reference to DRGs; and the hospital industry had to swallow the bitter pill in order to save face.

The DRG scenario does not fit the usual American pluralist model animated by civic interests approaching the state with demands and solutions, wherein the Congress responds by distributing benefits to each major interest group so that each gains a little and the status quo persists (Lowi 1979: 241–8). Rather the DRG programme represents the growing tendency to centralize authority at the federal level, a tendency abetted by the rise of a professional-bureaucratic complex. To cite Beer at some length:

> I would remark how rarely additions to the public sector have been initiated by the demands of voters or the advocacy of pressure groups or

the platforms of political parties. On the contrary, in the fields of health, housing, urban renewal, transportation, welfare, education, poverty, and energy it has been, in very great measure, people in government service, or closely associated with it, acting on the basis of their specialized knowledge, who first perceived the problem, conceived the programs, initially urged it to the President and Congress, went on to help lobby it through to enactment, and then saw to its administration. (1978: 423)

With Congressional prompting and support, HCFA proposed, developed, and implemented DRGs as a solution to controlling Medicare costs despite the opposition of providers. In the process, professional autonomy was curtailed. While the AMA and the AHA conducted their business as usual, HCFA officials quietly developed their own expertise over several years through involvement with the regional PSROs, the Yale University team which developed the DRGs, and the New Jersey State Health Department where experimental trials were conducted (Dunham and Marone 1984). Indeed, DRGs originally were developed through PSRO-related research efforts to assist in the development of norms and standards. As the mounting federal deficit plus economic pressure on the private business sector strengthened the resolve of key Congressional personnel to control Medicare costs, the opposing provider interests became more expendable. No private interest came forward with a viable alternative solution while HCFA and its professional associates were prepared with one.

Indeed, it may be stressed that, from a financing perspective, the DRG solution was not a radical one. It presents yet another incremental change from rate setting strategies of TEFRA and the earlier 1972 Social Security Act amendments, both of which contained forms of prospective reimbursement. But DRGs are special because they involve an all-inclusive payment rate per discharge which does not allow for add-ons. However, the political question is who has the power to determine the mechanism and the conditions under which it is operationalized. The answer is clearly HCFA, a federal agency which is in effect authorized by Congress to replace the traditional authority of the local hospitals to determine reimbursement rates. HCFA was ordered to devise a new mechanism for prospective finance as well as the standards on which it could be based. HCFA has emerged as a well-insulated bureaucratic agency with a public service mission and a formidable set of skills. The traditional health care providers, who have just as high a stake as HCFA, can no longer rely on support from their long-standing Congressional allies – especially because the Congress now has an obvious stake in cost containment. It is also probable that most members of Congress do not understand the complexities of the law they have passed, and therefore have left the real battles of implementation to be fought by others.

Peer review organizations, which are to monitor the application of DRGs, provide an equally compelling story about the simultaneous limitations on *and* expansion of professional power. After years of progressively limiting PSRO funding, HCFA had finally eliminated it altogether from the D/HSS programme budget. PSRO activities had not proved to be worth the costs of funding them (Lebish 1982: 996). However, the chairman of the Senate Finance Committee and other significant members were concerned about the 'quality aspect' of DRGs and were sympathetic to assuring the quality of care. At the chairman's prompting, HCFA created a second generation of PSROs, now called PROs or 'PSROs with teeth'. Compared with their PSRO predecessors, which were more or less federally chartered, quality assurance and utilization review activities are now contracted out to single state-wide physician-sponsored organizations.

More importantly, the transition from PSROs to PROs has been accompanied by a shift in guidance. PSROs were relatively independent of national standards, largely because they were provider dominated and fitted some aspects of the pluralistic model. The PSRO programme had delegated effective control to local physicians because the AMA had gone to the Congress, bargained for autonomous control, and received what it sought. The federal administrators served more or less routinely to approve decisions made at the local level; any state agency involvement was largely limited to educational activity.

However, PROs contrast with their predecessors in critical ways, particularly their dependence on HCFA for standards. Furthermore, the demand for continuing PSRO activities came from – in addition to the powerful Senate Finance Committee chairman – private groups and others without a major constituency. It was not the AMA which asked for their continuance; it was a subset of physicians who were in the business of reviewing their peers . . . or intervening on behalf of their peers, depending on how you look at it. PSROs had been starved for resources and were facing extinction. While Congress ensured that PSRO-like activities would continue, the solution really emerged from HCFA which once again stepped into the policy vacuum. HCFA's major ally or fellow-thinker was the American Medical Peer Review Associates – a group of physicians whose primary interest lay in evaluations and methodology.

HCFA established tight central control by contracting under stringent conditions determined by the federal agency's vision of the programme. These were then written into the law. Unlike utilization review or PSRO, programme authority was not simply delegated to private providers. The contracts contain measurable goals plus a promise (threat) by HCFA of non-renewal if the PROs do not meet expectations. In some sense, PROs now do have advantages for they will be better insulated than their predecessors. They also have accumulated significant resources to carry out the tasks, including the expertise developed over the years through PSRO review activities, the special knowledge required to review medical work, the necessary funds adequate to the task, the technological resources such as computers and associated software, and not least the power of the state to enforce their decisions. Given these resources plus the fact that physician groups had to bid for contracts and agree to their terms, it seems somewhat less likely than usual that the regulators (the PROs as HCFA agents) will be easily captured by the regulated (the local physicians and the hospitals through which they work).

In short, the state is no longer totally dependent on organized medicine for the special expertise required for trenchant review activities. HCFA not only has established norms and standards against which to measure medical practice. It also can rely on a faction of physicians, who do not represent a consensus of professional opinion, to enforce them (Boulanger 1984; Anderson and Shields 1982). HCFA may have learned the merit of a divide-and-rule strategy in a profession increasingly divided against itself. PROs certainly give those physicians who are ideologically sympathetic to centralized control of medicine an opportunity to practise their beliefs – with themselves at the controls! (This situation is not unlike the opportunity provided by HMO laws to physicians who desired group practice.) But it cannot and should not be assumed that PROs are monolithic or united in their intent.

Indeed, a less sanguine view can be taken of HCFA's ability to impose its authority directly through PROs and thereby limit the autonomous control of individual physicians over clinical decision-making. Large bureaucracies necessarily experience loss of information and loss of hierarchical control (Ostrom 1983). The structure of the PRO programme assumes that physician implementers – the PRO officials – have the same incentives as HCFA officials. For the programme to be successful, the structure assumes that local physicians will cooperate or can be forced to cooperate through threat of and/or application of sanctions. It further assumes that the power struggle between hospital administrators and physicians has been resolved.

Faced with the inevitable, AMA officials have encouraged

medical societies to make the best of an external review process and its limits on individual self-regulation. The AMA has encouraged state medical societies to bid on PRO contracts. But what does 'make the best' mean? Perhaps it means that some PRO physicians will remain protective of professional interests and act as a buffer between community physicians and the state, bending the rules in favour of local needs. Perhaps it means that some PRO physicians are not sympathetic at all to the PRO mission and will try to sabotage it. As a conduit for flows of information between the local physicians and the state, PROs will have ample opportunity for turning control toward their own ends. Whatever 'the best' means, it is not clear that PRO physicians will act as a cohesive cadre of HCFA agents.

In order to be effective, the PRO physicians must elicit the cooperation of local physicians – unless, under extreme circumstances, PROs are willing to disqualify large numbers of physicians from Medicare participation. But one outstanding revelation of PSRO-related research was the pervasive variation in clinical practice and the high degree of clinical uncertainty of which the variation is, in part, a result (Wennberg et al. 1982). Medicine remains more art than science, and patients and their clinical surroundings are more variable than had previously been realized – or at least acknowledged. Between two obvious and rather crude extremes of over- and underutilization there lies a discretionary range of medical judgement. The question is then once again raised as to what is the acceptable level of quality of care. What is the 'necessary margin of inappropriate use which must be tolerated in as complex an area as health care' (Anderson and Shields 1982: 132)? There is neither a consensus among experts as to what is an adequate volume of services, nor guidelines for most procedures.

But HCFA, like Congress, is interested in paying the least amount for care; it wants, as Eisenhower used to say, to obtain the most bang for the buck. The standards and norms which are the foundation for the payment and review systems have been developed in this context. The norms represent a bureaucratic judgement that the average amount of care is adequate. Indeed, the lowest possible use of services becomes the target. The norms themselves are statistical artifacts that may bear no resemblance to clinical efficacy but instead reflect the demands of the federal budget.

Conflict between PROs and the physicians will be over the acceptability to physicians of the norms that the PROs must enforce. The physician acts as the patient's agent in ordering care which he/she provides to the individual according to a patient-centred ethic and under conditions of uncertainty. On the other hand, providing care according to externally imposed standards requires that the clinician act indirectly as HCFA's agent rather than solely as the patient's agent. This conflict of interest centres on the physician's traditional role in which he/she exercises autonomous clinical judgement. We have returned to the heart of a profession (Freidson 1970: 83–4).

Consequently, recast in political terms, the conflict over norms and standards is a conflict of claims between two camps of experts. One set of experts – who are experts in cost containment and resource management – demands the right to determine the norms because it holds the purse strings and has the power of the state behind it. The other set of experts – the heterogeneous group of practising physicians – demands the professional right to practise according to internalized norms, transmitted to them through education, precept and practice, because they are the trained professionals and because they have the patients. In sum, the conflict between HCFA agent and patient agent will be played out in the battle over norms. Since there is no 'ideal type' of medical model which absolutely maximizes health, and since the pluralistic political model is likely to continue in the US, the outcomes will necessarily reflect a compromise among professional, financial and – not least – patient expectations. However, whatever autonomy physicians lose will be absorbed by HCFA and its PRO agents, as representatives of the state. Authority, once delegated to doctors via autonomy and monopoly, may be returning to its point of origin.

Finally, to carry the bureaucratic logic one step further, HCFA will require a monitoring mechanism – a super-PRO – to monitor the PROs and to ensure that they are acting faithfully. Such a super-PRO would present two countervailing forces; one would tighten HCFA control through another insulated layer of expertise in the areas of utilization review and quality assurance, while the other would weaken HCFA control through yet another bureaucratic layer of officials with their own interests. If HCFA is not successful in containing costs – which requires, fundamentally, changing physician behaviour – then questions will emerge about the cost effectiveness of its DRG and PRO programmes. However, as the history of PSROs has shown, once organizations infiltrate the political system, they somehow find the means to sustain themselves. Controlling physician behaviour seems to be a lucrative occupation.

It might also be noted in passing that, among other things, computers made DRGs possible (Robinson 1982; Dudley 1984). The case-mix data necessary for managing DRGs provide administrators with information about the practice patterns of each physician. Combined with the incentive to use the information, this is sufficient for the administrator to try to influence the medical staff in order to alter their practice patterns in favour of the hospital (Lebish 1982: 991–8). This means that physicians will be asked to force a fit between their practice patterns and the practice norms established by HCFA. And computers will keep track of the points – game, set and match!

Summary, Conclusions, and Reflections

Since 1965 the American federal government has moved increment-ally through a series of programmes which have progressively encroached upon the professional prerogatives of physicians in terms of their technical autonomy. This intrusion began with utiliza-tion review (UR) which did not, in effect, limit technical autonomy. However, for the first time organized medicine was put on notice by its long-standing allies in Congress that technical autonomy was fair game for administrative review. Also, UR brought about the development of a hospital committee infrastructure for a physician practice review system that grew through PSROs and persists in the DRGs monitored by PROs.

When UR failed to contain costs, Congress developed a more extensive solution through the professional standards review organ-izations programme. Three of the five major categories of patient care management variables were brought under review, and data were aggregated to permit the development of standards and norms against which physician practice patterns could be measured. An unanticipated result of the research efforts to help the PSROs develop norms and standards was the appearance of diagnostic-related groups (DRGs). Throughout the era of UR and PSRO, the constraint of insufficient knowledge of what constitutes an accept-able level of quality in care resulted in an inability to assess a reasonable trade-off between cost and quality.

Nonetheless, fiscal exigencies required drastic action. Cost cutting measures were undertaken in the form of DRGs which use averages derived from Medicare billing data as a proxy of reasonable cost and, by implication, reasonable quality of care. PSROs were replaced by the utilization and quality control peer review organization (PRO) programme, the latter having much greater power to penalize providers. PROs are better insulated against local forces, and they account for the full range of clinical management variables. Unlike PSROs, which relied on the hospital committees to perform review activities, PROs send their own employees into the hospital in order to conduct their own more stringent reviews. Since PSRO-like activities are also being maintained within the hospitals' utilization review and quality assurance committees, the new DRG committees have been added to a lengthening list of committees reviewing physician practice patterns.

In 1965 physicians were practising medicine with almost complete technical autonomy over clinical decisions. Now the fears expressed by outraged physicians in response to the 1972 PSRO programme seem to have been well founded in political reality. The quasi-governmental penetration into the realm of physician practice patterns has been substantial with the development of norms and standards based on averages. Physician practice patterns with costs repeatedly above the average are assumed to represent over-utilization of resources and therefore unnecessary care. Since the overriding objective of PROs and DRGs is cost containment, these changes mirror the fears of physicians about where PSROs would lead. The government's promise of non-interference with medical practice that enveloped the spirit of the 1965 Medicare law was inevitably undermined by the fact that utilization review was part of that legislation. The cost containment imperative is the driving force behind the government's incursion into medicine, and controlling the technical autonomy of physicians is its lever over costs.

Despite all this, physicians still have an escape hatch. Just as hospital administrators engage in cost shifting, physicians can switch from in-patient service to provide more care in their unregulated out-patient settings. This in fact already appears to be occurring. The AMA prints a unified health insurance claim form as a for-profit service to physicians (who can purchase them at a discount) and a variety of third-party payers. Demand for out-patient forms has increased exponentially since DRG regulation was implemented (Marone and Dunham 1984). It may be a mistake, however, to assume that physicians and hospitals will continue to have this safety valve. DRGs and PROs constitute a sizeable increment, if not a leap, in government surveillance of medical practice patterns. Of course, organized medicine has an impressive historical record of parrying and deflecting proposals which would undermine its professional autonomy and control. Indeed it is important to remember that the DRG legislation initially contained a provision that would have mandated prospective pricing for physician fees, an omission from the final legislation which was a concession to the AMA. But HCFA is in the process of developing DRG-like fixed payment rules for out-patient medical services as well. Given the cost containment imperative, areas where physicians can exercise professional prerogatives – such as out-patient services for piece-work fees – are a prime target for further regulation.

It is sometimes said that any doctor worth his degree can beat the system. DRGs and any additional stringent regulation of out-patient fees will seriously test this proposition. The danger is that physicians will try to evade each governmental effort aimed at limiting their autonomy, which may provoke both parties to engage in an extended regulatory battle for control over medical resources until the goal of rationalizing physician behaviour overwhelms any remaining concerns for quality and access. The regulatory path from UR to DRGs is clearly marked both by government attempts to apply increasingly stringent controls to physician autonomy, and by physicians' attempts to evade those controls.

The United States is currently attempting two simultaneous but contradictory approaches to the problems of the health sector. One is its traditional preference for pluralism; the other is the siren song of an orderly imposition of centralized standards. A pluralistic system in which change is made incrementally is self-correcting; it is meliorative since it fixes what went wrong or attends to issues formerly not considered as interest groups make their demands known to policy-makers. But could a pluralistic political system moved by incremental decision-making lead to a health care system suffocated under a quagmire of regulations that are insensitive to concerns for quality and access? Can cost be controlled while quality and access are retained and even enhanced? The current answer seems to be: 'Let's try.'

Because of the complexity and high degree of specialized knowledge required to understand the cost containment problem and its associated trade-offs, this task has been handed over by Congress to the bureaucracy. HCFA has obtained an enormous amount of power to make decisions in this area, but bureaucracy tends by its very nature to impose solutions. Furthermore, bureaucracy generally has not been known for its permeability to public concerns or to organized interests not already aligned with its official and unofficial goals. The question is whether the American health care system now remains sufficiently pluralistic for the self-correcting effects associated with pluralism to occur, or whether the constriction wrought by the newly empowered bureaucracy will so centralize the system that it eventually crumbles under its own weight. Until the present, the autonomy of physicians had accounted, in large part, for both the flexibility in the health system and the gigantic national health care bill. The question is: what next?

To return to more general themes, politicizing medicine is a reasonably clear process in the US and elsewhere. Some might observe that medicine has always been political in several senses. Certainly physicians have always wielded power in the sense of advising, directing, and sometimes changing the behaviour of patients. Also physicians have historically organized and fought to retain self-regulation and the existence of a private government with internal controls over membership. But most clearly of all, medicine has been politicized as the public and its governments have sought to control and regulate the behaviour of physicians – and as these physicians and their organizations have fought back with counter-measures including lobbying, publicizing, proselytizing and cam-paigning in overt politics.

More problematic is the concept of 'medicalizing politics', but the evidence accumulates on at least two fronts. First, there is simply the quantity or proportion of politics and political activity that is devoted to medical matters. Almost every major newspaper as well as broadcast journalism contains daily reports on health politics from local issues through national concerns. The activities of politicized medicine (or 'organized medicine' as some would put it) contribute to this increasing proportion of medical issues among the general issues of public debate. If measured in the passage, repassage, and refinement of laws alone and the time spent debating them in legislative chambers and executive corridors, there is ample evidence that medical affairs have entered the very substance of politics. Likewise the literally volumes of regulations and guidelines on health care that are proposed, revised, finalized and published attest to the medicalization of politics.

Secondly, however, politics has been medicalized in an even larger philosophical sense. As the American health care crisis has become chronic, it has generated an impressive array of palliative reforms, for example: equal access; improved quality; cost contain-ment; consumer participation; ethics committees; and preventive health. At the same time, the hegemony of the therapeutic ideology articulated by the helping professions has steadily increased. Each reform contributes to this hegemony. For example, achieving equal access broadens the clientele of medicine while establishing medical service as a legal right. Ensuring quality care intensifies popular beliefs that professionals know what care is. Cost control assures not health but a rationalized guarantee of the medical system's income. Consumer participation coopts potentially disruptive citi-zens by providing participation in medical matters as a substitute for political action. Ethical issues expand medical hegemony by con-cluding that issues like abortion and life prolongation are medical questions. And preventive health can make every person a patient each day of his/her life. 'Each reform, therefore, represents a new opportunity for the medical system to expand its influence, scale and control' (McKnight 1975: 5).

The political functions of this chronic health care crisis may be obvious but merit reiteration. As new needs are created by expanding alternative medical systems, citizens develop an increased sense of deficiency and dependence. As dependency grows, so do medical resources devoted to 'curing' the health problems. Likewise, political energies are increasingly consumed in efforts to reform the medical system. Yet the growth of medicalized politics induces a further popular acceptance of expertise. People act less as citizens and more like clients, that is those people who believe they will be better because someone else knows better. Viewed in these terms, the medicalization of politics involves the propagation of a therapeutic ideology; only the professional few understand, so medicine becomes the paradigm for modernized domination (Edelman 1974; Ehrenreich 1978).

But what about physician power *per se*? What about the frequent assertion – so frequent, in fact, that it has almost become folklore – that doctors dominate the health system and always receive the most benefits? In the United States at least, organized medicine – while unable to prevent some major legislation – has been able to use the power of withdrawing its labour (vital to society by virtue of professional expertise) in order to obtain substantial concessions based on aspects of professionalism. The AMA has been able to retain vital levers of control through concessions claimed on the grounds of professionalism. Of course, things aren't as easy as they used to be. In 1934 a quiet word persuaded the House Ways and Means Committee to drop even its directive to the proposed social security board to study the matter of national health insurance. But while the failure of organized medicine to prevent the Medicare and Medicaid legislation in 1965 may be seen as a decline in its power, 'the provision for paying doctors under part B of Medicare reflected the legislators' fears that doctors would act on their repeated threats of non-cooperation in implementing Medicare.' Thus no fee schedule was prescribed and the doctors of Medicare patients were to be paid their usual and customary fee (Dyckman 1978). The professional claim to demand fees for service – a major aspect of the status (and hence power) of professionalism – was preserved by the fact that 'it was not required that the doctor directly charge the insurance company intermediaries who were to handle the government payments; he could bill the patient, who, after paying his debt, would be reimbursed by the insurance company' (Marmor 1976: 81).

The claim that physicians control the health sector, therefore, requires some modification. In so far as they retain and exercise major aspects of professionalism, they control vital aspects of the health sector. But the extent to which these aspects add up to total control of health services varies. Certainly many features of professionalism are under challenge. The professional right to define health itself has been disputed by alternative formulations, not to mention the overall dilemma for medical dominance posed by the persistent problem of escalating health costs. Control over the supply and number of doctors available is also increasingly subject to political rather than professional decisions. The increase in the number of doctors has been the result of governmental response to public expectations of more and better health facilities. The fears of a doctor surplus on the part of organized medicine reflects not professional control (or means of control), but professional concern in the face of the political decision to cut back in all fields of public expenditure. Finally the latitude of physicians to determine the acceptable range of fees for service is slowly lessening; technical autonomy, upon which professional power is founded, is being eroded by information retrieval and refined computational capacities.

Apart from these constraints, the medical profession in the United States would appear to have retained a sufficient number of the characteristics of professionalism to be said to dominate the health sector, if not completely control it. In matters of cost, peer review, health planning and resource allocation, the American profession remains well placed owing to the continued pluralistic structure of the health system.

One final point might be made about the power of physicians in the United States and the growing constraints being placed upon it. Clearly medicine is politicized, while politics has a very large and increasing component of medical care issues within its ambit. But the obvious point – perhaps so obvious that it is sometimes overlooked – is the evident American willingness to use state power to address a social and economic dilemma. The sequential existence of UR committees, PSROs and PROs/DRGs, with their impact on technical autonomy and physician practice patterns, is all the more remarkable because Americans generally dislike power (or, as Anthony King once quipped, like it so much they don't want anyone else to have any) and try to limit it through the classical separation of powers and complicated intergovernmental relations. Evidently there is still a pioneering spirit, a brashness in action, a sense of 'can do' and 'fix it' rather than fatalistically accepting things as they are. In the US, politicized medicine and medicalized politics seem to add up to a slow but inevitable diminution of physician power.

As an afterthought to stimulate comparative inquiry and debate, perhaps European states have not been as aggressive in attempting to control their professionals of the medical persuasion because the

United States has always existed as an exit option (Hirschman 1970) for the latter's practice of medicine. Given its preponderant economic size and relatively permeable boundaries, the American economy has served from a distance to shape governmental policies about the health sector in Europe. Certainly this point seems true of the United Kingdom in so far as the most outspoken critics of state medicine are those British doctors who have come to the 'freedom of the States' in order to get away from the bureaucracy of socialized medicine. There have been many fewer articulate spokesmen or advocates of the National Health Service available *in* the US speaking out on behalf of greater state control of this otherwise 'private government' called the American health (non-) system. Thus, while European states have attempted structurally to control physicians through the appointment and deployment of personnel, the centralization of finances and even influencing the preparatory curricula, they have not disciplined practitioners by monitoring their technical practice (and thus challenging their autonomy) for fear they would leave. Now that the US has acted, however, the exit option has been constricted – though not, of course, altogether eliminated. Thus the alternative option of giving voice (if not loyalty) has appeared wherein government policies are implemented to control the powerful medical profession.

3

Health Professionals
in the Swedish System

Jan-Erik Lane and Sven Arvidson

In the welfare state the provision of health in various forms is a task for different kinds of professionals: people trained in various disciplines in accordance with defined curricula, examined in terms of institutionalized criteria, and legitimized by adherence to precise procedures. Without core groups of health professionals no modern system of health care could operate, but the organizational structures in which these professionals work may vary. Two fundamental alternatives may be identified: market systems versus public resource allocation systems on the one hand, and centralized versus decentralized forms of public systems on the other. Some nations combine market and public resource allocation, whereas others primarily trust one of these mechanisms of allocation. In public systems of health care provision the allocation of resources may be centralized by the state or it may be entrusted to some organizational unit at another level of government, such as the local government system.

The choice of basic system has an impact on health professionals. It may be argued that their autonomy or power will be larger in a market-oriented system than in a public system; but what of a centralized versus a decentralized system in a predominantly public system of health resource allocation? The development of the Swedish system of health care is interesting from this systemic point of view: is decentralization conducive to professional autonomy? In order to illuminate the relation between the position of health professionals and the issue of centralization, an analysis of trends towards decentralization in the Swedish system offers some interesting clues. Is it to be taken for granted that organizational decentralization must result in greater professional autonomy?

Public Sector Expansion

In Sweden there has been an expansion of the public sector as well as an effort to decentralize. There was formerly an active private health care system with numerous independent practitioners and private hospitals. However, the expansion of the welfare state has transformed the local government system into an almost monopoly supplier of health care. At the same time the market for health care services has been closely regulated by a fixed system of remuneration. Since 1955 the state has paid part of the bill by means of insurance.

The rise of the county councils as the main provider of health care is conspicuous. The 23 county councils and the few municipalities outside the county council system allocated in 1960 about 2.3 percent of the GNP, in 1970 4.6 percent, and in 1982 no less than 11.4 percent. Roughly 85 percent of their budgets is allocated to health care. Their function as a regional employer is matched by few private firms. In 1960 there were 136,000 employees in the county councils; by 1986 this had risen to 417,840, mostly women. More than four-fifths of the employees within the health system are employed by county councils. As a result of this process of public resource allocation expansion, only vestiges of the private system remain.

The organizational development of the county councils is a combination of an expansion of volume and a transfer of tasks from the state and the private sector to this regional part of the local government sector. In 1928 the county councils were obliged to supply in-patient health care. Nation-wide planning was initiated in 1958 when the counties were divided into health care regions. In 1959 responsibility for hospital out-patient care was also placed with

Table 3.1 *Health care consumption in Sweden 1970–85*
(in real economic terms: million Swedish kronor at 1985 prices)

	1970	1975	1980	1985	Change 1970–85 (%)
Private consumption	6,444	5,958	6,118	7,155	11
As percentage of GDP	1.0	0.8	0.8	0.8	
Public consumption	30,196	43,984	58,936	61,794	104
As percentage of GNP	4.8	5.8	7.3	7.2	
Public subsidies to					
Medical drugs	1,914	3,228	3,582	3,830	100
Private physicians					
and dentists	646	2,588	2,840	2,462	281
Total health					
consumption	39,200	55,759	71,476	75,241	92
As percentage of GDP	6.2	7.4	8.8	8.7	35

Source: Hälsostatistisk Årsbok 1987/88: Table D. 19: 112

the county councils. The open health care system outside hospitals was transferred to the county councils in 1963, and psychiatric care in 1967.

Typical of the Swedish system of health care is its public orientation. In addition, whereas the proportion of GNP allocated to health care is about the same in Sweden as in similar rich countries, its health care programmes are more oriented towards hospital care. Table 3.1 (p. 75) shows the process of cost expansion compared with the growth of GNP. It also indicates the process of growth of public control.

The private health care sector is smaller in Sweden than in other similar Western nations. The incidence of health care inside and outside hospitals distinguishes Sweden, which has a much heavier emphasis on hospital care than most other countries (Table 3.2).

Table 3.2   *Number of visits to doctors in Sweden (millions)*

	Public				Public and Private	
	At hospitals	Outside hospitals	Total	Private	Total	Per person
1960	5.6	NA	NA	NA	15.3	2.0
1970	8.8	5.6	14.4	4.8	19.2	2.4
1973	9.3	6.3	15.7	4.3	20.0	2.5
1976	10.4	7.0	17.4	3.6	21.0	2.6
1977	10.7	7.4	18.1	3.4[1]	21.5	2.6
1984	10.4	11.4	21.8	2.8	24.6	2.9

NA: No statistics available.
[1]Estimated value.

Source: SOU 1981:2:141

Hospital treatment basically consists of three kinds of care. Somatic short-term treatment is distinguished from somatic long-term treatment, both of which are separated from psychiatric care. The relative size of these basic modes has changed over time (Table 3.3). The amount of resources allocated to somatic long-term treatment has greatly increased while the number of nursing places in the two traditional types of hospital care has gone down. A combination of demographic changes, technological innovations and political measures explains these trends. In the past decade, national health care planning has attempted to transfer resources from in-patient to out-patient health care. So-called primary care has been expanded but not as much as the central authorities wished.

Table 3.3   *Numbers of beds in in-patient care in Sweden 1960–84*

Nursing places	1960	1970	1975	1977	1985
Somatic short term	50,300	49,400	47,100	46,300	36,900
Somatic long term	18,600	33,600	40,300	41,800	51,500
Psychiatric care	34,500	37,000	36,300	34,500	20,900
Total	103,400	120,000	123,700	122,600	114,200

Sources: SOU 1981:2:124; *Hälsostatistisk Årsbok* 1987/88

The county councils provide about half of Sweden's dental care, the other half being private but regulated in detail. The national dental care service was introduced in 1938 and has been expanded into a general system for dental care for all children up to 19 years of age. County council dental care also covers specialist treatment and voluntary care for adults.

The growing emphasis on public control in Sweden's health care system has had profound implications for its health professionals. Almost all of them are now public employees and their trade unions relate to public sector employers' associations. As Table 3.4 indicates, the degree of organization among the health professionals is high.

Table 3.4   *Trade unions of health professionals in Sweden: membership and public employment 1983[1]*

	Läkarförbundet[2]	Tandläkarförbundet[3]	SHSTF[4]	LSR[5]
Total number of members	21,200	10,500	70,000	6,211
Members publicly employed	17,500	7,000	67,200	4,037
Percentage	82.5	66.7	96.0	65.0

[1] More than 80 percent of those publicly employed are employed by the county councils. In addition to the four trade unions which organize health professionals, there are others that organize other categories of employees in the health system. The great bulk of unskilled health workers are organized in the Svenska Kommunalarbetareförbundet (SKAF). The trade unions of the health professionals organize about 95 percent of their possible members.

[2] The Swedish Medical Association, which organizes the physicians.

[3] Tandläkarförbundet organizes the dentists.

[4] The SHSTF organizes categories like trained nurses, ward sisters and midwives.

[5] The LSR is the trade union of the physiotherapists.

Source: Interviews and correspondence with the trade unions

There are some basic distinctions among health professionals. One line of separation is between academic professionals and non-academic professionals. Another line of separation divides state employees and local government employees. As stated above, the role of the state as employer has been reduced. Health professionals are centred in one type of public organization, the regional local government tier of the county councils. There are 23 county councils which, in addition to three major municipalities, carry out health care functions.

County Council Organizational Growth

The county councils were previously rather small organizations, run by laymen and a small administrative staff. The process of expanding the public provision of health services has been accompanied by a process of bureaucratization. Currently the county councils contain a sizeable administrative staff at various levels. Indeed the administrative component of the county councils has developed its own planning and coordination techniques which can challenge overall national planning.

Two types of administrative staff exist within the county councils. On the one hand, there is the central administrative body close to the political machinery of the county councils. Data indicate that the size of this central administrative body has expanded more rapidly than overall operations. By distinguishing between the huge county council of Stockholm with its own accounting system and the remaining county councils, Table 3.5 presents information about this development of bureaucratization. The costs for the central administrative body have expanded from roughly 1.5 percent of the total cost to about 2.5 percent since the early 1960s. As the absolute increase in the overall operations of the county councils is sevenfold – from 1.4 billion to almost 10 billion Swedish crowns – there has been a considerable expansion in administration.

On the other hand, we must also take into account the administrative resources that are more closely connected with ongoing operations. Each hospital has an administrative structure, and varieties of administrative personnel are in close contact with the various clinics. Table 3.6 shows the development of staff in the county councils. Included in the set of administrative staff are the personnel of the central administrative body. As the county councils developed into major regional employers – from 154,000 full-time jobs in 1974 to 227,000 full-time jobs in 1981 – the administrative component expanded marginally. In 1974 it constituted about 8

Table 3.5 *County councils in Sweden: costs and administrative costs per capita 1950–82 (Swedish crowns: 1983 prices)*

	1950	1954	1958	1962	1966	1970	1974	1978	1982
All except Stockholm[1]									
Total	582	817	1,060	1,452	2,373	3,870	6,008	9,038	9,853
Central administration	9	15	15	22	51	97	147	220	252
Percentage	1.57	1.78	1.37	1.52	2.16	2.50	2.43	2.42	2.54
Stockholm council									
Total	658	912	1,370	1,738	2,742	3,841	7,442	10,004	11,817
Central administration	16	35	19	34	112	190	470	674	304
Percentage	2.43	3.84	1.39	1.96	4.08	4.95	6.32	6.74	2.57[2]

[1] Average per council.
[2] The decreasing cost is due to changes in organization.

Source: Kommunernas finanser 1950–82

Table 3.6   *County councils in Sweden: numbers of full-time employees and administrative staff 1973–83*

	1973	1974	1975	1976	1977	1978	1979	1980	1981	1982	1983
All except Stockholm[1]											
Total	6,567	6,988	7,189	7,799	8,259	8,957	9,447	9,933	10,322	10,504	10,888
Administrative staff	534	569	591	659	711	783	839	878	907	925	962
Percentage	8.05	8.07	8.14	8.36	8.56	8.69	8.84	8.77	8.74	8.76	8.78
Stockholm council											
Total	34,750	39,168	40,568	42,605	44,653	48,380	51,211	52,931	56,380	63,470	64,937
Administrative staff	4,079	5,019	4,693	5,012	5,320	5,559	5,961	6,086	6,221	7,204	7,537
Percentage	11.74	12.81	11.57	11.76	11.91	11.49	11.64	11.50	11.03	11.35	11.61

[1] Average per council.

Source: Landstingsförbundet (1973–83)

percent whereas in 1981 it made up 9 percent of full-time jobs (except the county council of Stockholm).

Notwithstanding the process of bureaucratization in the county councils, the bulk of those employed in the county councils are health professionals. The relative proportions of various kinds of professional staff are shown in Table 3.7.

Health Professionals and the Public Structure

The power of health professionals is a function of how they relate to central government as well as to local government, and of how they relate to each other. The capacity of professionals to take decisions and implement actions concerning the provision of health in Sweden depends on their relationships with public organizations, mainly the county councils (including three municipalities) as well as central government bodies involved in health care provision. The autonomy of health professionals depends on how much autonomy the county councils have in relation to the state as well as on how much power the professionals are able to secure for themselves within the county council system.

The formal organization of intergovernmental relations is contradictory, as it is based on a tension between two legal principles. One is the constitutionally guaranteed rule that a local government may take care of its own affairs. The other is the general principle of parliamentary legislative power: that is, central government may introduce directives as to *what* the county councils should do (primary autonomy) as well as to *how* they should do it (secondary autonomy). Thus, the county councils enjoy a broad taxation power to pay for a large programme structure involving educational, cultural and sports activities as well as health care.

However, the central government governs these activities in various ways. From 1962 there existed a detailed system of rules that restricted the discretion of the county councils with regard to both what they might do and how they might go about doing it. Basically, a distinction may be made between two kinds of these legal restrictions. On the one hand, there was legislation which obliged health care organizations to take measures to provide publicly for basic services in this area. The health care law was the core of the directives laid down by the centre as to how regional organizations were to handle the provision of health care. The set of central directives included accompanying laws as well as bureaucratic norms. On the other hand, there existed a set of legal interpretations of the nature of the discretion involved in the autonomy clause 'to handle their own affairs'. National adminis-

Table 3.7 *Full-time employees in all 23 Swedish county councils in health care and administration, 1973, 1978, 1983*

	1973		1978		1983		Percentage change 1973–83
	Number	Percent	Number	Percent	Number	Percent	
Total full-time employees	179,218	100.0	245,434	100.0	304,481	100.0	+70
Physicians	6,371	4.0	10,590	4.3	14,932	4.9	+134
Dentists	2,451	1.4	2,855	1.2	3,942	1.3	+61
Trained nurses	21,606	12.0	28,030	11.0	38,613	12.5	+79
Ward sisters	6,217	3.0	8,461	3.0	10,492	3.4	+69
Dental nurses	3,438	1.9	5,164	2.1	7,989	2.6	+132
Physiotherapists	1,440	0.8	2,168	0.8	2,872	0.9	+99
Nurses' assistants	72,733	40.6	98,000	39.9	111,959	36.8	+54
Dental nurses' assistants	168	0.1	512	0.2	1,121	0.4	+567
Administrative staff	15,827	8.8	22,785	9.3	28,701	9.4	+81
Other categories	48,967	27.3	66,869	27.2	83,860	27.5	+71

Source: Landstingsförbundet (1973, 1978, 1983)

trative court decisions interpreted the legal implications of the principle of 'their own affairs'.

As a result of these two sets of very different legal restrictions the county councils previously did not possess far-reaching discretion. Their financial and organizational status was not matched by institutional autonomy. The discrepancy between economic resources and power was the chief source of the growing demand for the regionalization of the health care system, manifested in the 1982 legislation increasing county council discretion. There is also quite substantial central government support for the drive towards regionalization, partly as a result of the state financial crisis which began in 1976.

The state has been much more involved in the output of the county councils than in the input of resources. About 60 percent of the resources of the county councils is derived from the county council tax. Roughly 20 percent comes from the state in the form of various grants, about 10 percent is derived from charges and another 10 percent stems from various other sources including borrowing.

In such a basically public structure for the provision of health care the situation of the health professionals – their autonomy in relation to their responsibility for health care, and their capacity to influence what other bodies decide – is conditioned by two different sources of directives: national government and local government. Correspondingly, it is possible to identify two distinct models of governance in the area of health care provision: a centralized system and a decentralized system. The extent to which the national legal framework delimits the autonomy of the county councils depends on the structure of the legal system. In 1982 a revision of the legal framework was introduced, based on a reconsideration of the relationship between the state and the county councils. The preceding legal framework based on 1962 legislation expressed a quite different model of state–county interaction from that implied in the 1982 legislation.

The State Model

The 1962 system (Sjukvårdslagen 1962: 242, Sjukvårdskungörelsen 1972: 676, Folktandvårdslagen 1973: 547, Folktandvårdskungörelsen 1973: 637) was oriented towards detailed regulation and close supervision. The main parliamentary law contained 36 paragraphs, augmented by 39 paragraphs in the supplemented government directives. These 75 rules not only laid down comprehensive duties on the part of the county councils to provide for hospital care but also specified in great detail how this general duty was to be carried out. Thus, the 1962 framework stated what hospital care amounted to, how the county council was to govern hospital care, and how the county council administration was to be structured. Moreover, the position and duties of the doctors were minutely regulated, the law distinguishing between various kinds of physicians and identifying their various responsibilities. Rules governed the conduct of hospital care, including the admission of patients, the recruitment of doctors, the treatment of patients and their release from hospital. The pre-1982 relationship between the state and the county councils was certainly not one of strong local government autonomy.

State control of county councils
Given the strong emphasis on hospital care in the Swedish system of health care, two factors were of central importance for the development of the system: the building of hospitals and the recruitment of physicians. In the 1962 system the centre exercised considerable control over these two decision parameters. Until 1982 the county council had to apply to the central authorities, mainly the Board for Health and Welfare. Central scrutiny was close and concerned both medical and financial aspects. The supply of doctors had a large impact on the county councils because formerly a severe shortage hampered county council developmental plans. The centre controlled the supply of physicians in two ways: on the one hand the centre determined the number of physicians examined each year, including what kinds of physicians the public education system produced; on the other hand the centre had to approve the requests of the various county councils for establishing new positions. Whereas the centre still controls the training of physicians, it no longer regulates the introduction of positions as physicians. The regional distribution of physicians is the outcome of a process of negotiation wherein each single county council (municipality) makes its own decisions.

It should be emphasized that the control exercised in the 1962 system but abolished in 1982 was of a passive nature. The centre waited for initiatives from the county councils about investment in capital and personnel, which the centre then examined and approved or denied. There was no active control through which the centre directed the county councils how to expand their budgets by centrally conceived initiatives. The removal of the central control over buildings and physicians has not meant that all mechanisms of central influence on county councils have been abolished. But the previous shortage of physicians has been transformed into a more balanced supply, and the period of large-scale investments in hospital buildings has come to an end.

The National Board of Health and Welfare had a general right to supervise the county councils: 'Fifth paragraph: the supreme duty to supervise the provision of health care by the county councils rests with the Board of Health and Welfare.' This general supervisory role of the centre in relation to county council health provision has been retained in the 1982 system (paragraph 18) but practice is different. Whereas the Board used to conduct numerous inspections, they are now less frequent.

State control of health professionals
Even though the centre no longer controls decisions about new investments and new positions, it still exercises a kind of review influence over the activities of the health professionals. There is a central agency – the Health and Medical Services Disciplinary Board – that enforces certain rules that protect against malpractice. As previously, the state exerts control over the public provision of health by means of a review process involving the possibility of legal action against malpractice. According to the so-called Lex Maria, the chief administrator of the county councils was under obligation to bring cases of malpractice to the attention of the Board of Health and Welfare as well as of the police in order that legal action be initiated. Besides the severe threat to a practitioner of a court examining a possible occurrence of malpractice, each and every patient could file a complaint with the central agency which had the power to issue a statement against the practitioner. If several such statements were made the practitioner would be prohibited from practice.

It should be emphasized that these central instruments of review were effective in establishing national rules of conduct in the provision of health care. Although there were few cases of legal action under the Lex Maria and although few practitioners had several statements lodged against them, the possibility of such severe sanctions was no doubt a strong threat. These review functions have not diminished in the 1982 system. The new rules replacing Lex Maria (Tillsynslagen 1982) strengthen and widen central audit functions.

The Local Government Model

The response to the expansion of health care services by the county councils has been planning. Each county council has a five-year planning system integrating the annual budget plans. Five-year planning documents developed during the 1970s. There was no legal regulation of these plans, but the introduction of planning was guided by norms developed by the Federation of Swedish County Councils – the Landstingsförbundet. The national association of county councils is a heavily staffed interest organization operating at the centre as a representative of the county councils; it negotiates with the state and participates in the national policy process. The Landstingsförbundet in collaboration with the National Board of Health and Welfare conducts long-term planning on the basis of the planning documents of the county councils (LKELP system). Moreover, the federation issues a large number of recommendations to the county councils in order to standardize their patterns of operations. Often these recommendations have been negotiated with the central bureaucracy.

The emergence of health care planning was typical of the 1970s as more and more health care activities were added to county council planning in accordance with norms and criteria recommended by the Federation, the central bureaucracy, and the semi-public Institute for Health Planning and Rationalization (SPRI). Two-thirds of SPRI is owned by the county councils and one-third by the state. It operates basically as a consultant in questions concerning rational, effective, and methodical development of health care.

The revision of the legal framework defining the role of the county councils in relation to the state may be interpreted in the light of the trends described above. The continuous expansion of the county councils has been accompanied by a growing demand for decentralization. The 1982 Health Act attempted such a reorientation. The large number of rules in the 1962 system is replaced by a small number of paragraphs stating the overall objectives of the health care system as well as outlining the main organizational structure of the system. Detailed central regulation and close supervision is to be replaced by broad planning and coordination of the central authorities.

The county councils are to be responsible not only for hospital care but also for the overall health of their inhabitants. The county councils are to structure the health provision in order to:

1   Satisfy the needs of patients for safety and quality of health care
2   Provide a comprehensive approach to conditions for the patient
3   Provide health care that is close to the patient as well as readily accessible, equal for all, with quality assured
4   Respect the rights of the individual to self-determination, integrity and relevant medical information.

Although the 1982 framework contains rules concerning the organization of the health care system as well as the conduct of health care itself, its emphasis is on influencing the county councils by means of general goals. Thus decentralization is to be combined with goal governance, and these replace the 1962 system with its centralization and rule governance. Detailed regulation, close supervision and careful control were typical of the centralized model, whereas planning is to be the mechanism for steering the county councils in the future. The planning system of the county councils is to be integrated in a national planning system.

The state now relies on two means of directing the activities of the county councils: by giving special grants for the kinds of health programmes it wishes to see in the county council budget; and by framing special conditions in the state insurance system which make the county councils more interested in certain programmes. Both of these influence mechanisms have been employed for various purposes. State grants have been channelled to psychiatric care as well as preventive care, whereas the insurance system has been employed to subsidize the provision of open health care. Although the county councils have never been highly dependent on state funding, state money still matters at the margin.

Health Care and Public Resource Allocation

The basic transformation of the relationships between central authorities and the county councils under the ideal of decentralization amounts to a shift from *control* to *negotiation*. A large set of central directives is replaced by central coordination and negotiations between the national government and the county councils (plus the three municipalities).

The central planning system involves the Riksdag and the government which are responsible for the identification of overall goals. The special Delegation for Health Care within the Ministry of Social Affairs is the chief planning body; it consists of politicians, bureaucrats, and representatives of the Landstingsförbundet. The central authorities publish planning documents regularly. These documents screen a number of aspects of the health care system on the basis of commissioned investigations about the existing situation and attempts at innovation. Thus far it is no exaggeration to claim that the main reports – *Health Care in the Eighties* by the Board, and *Health Care in the Nineties* by the Delegation – have played a role in determining the plans of the county councils. Although only recommendations about future developments in the health care system, these reports have an impact on the yearly decisions of the county councils through their influence on the five-year planning documents.

Even though the National Board of Health and Welfare was reorganized in the early 1980s, it remains an important bureau exercising supervision over the county councils. However, as the amount of detailed regulation has been reduced sharply, the functions of the Board are being reoriented toward planning. Thus, an official document states:

> It devolves upon the Board to take care of matters relating to national planning, considering the needs of individuals, the requirements of coordination and the supply of educated personnel, as well as to support regional and local planning. (SOU 1979: 78:159–60)

The role of the Board has declined as a result of the change from detailed supervision by the centre to coordination and negotiation. The standard description of the central planning system is one of harmony among the central authorities, the Landstingsförbundet and SPRI. Although there have been no major divergences in the principal documents of these central planning bodies, the future may see clashes between the state on the one hand and the county council executives on the other.

A number of central agencies besides the Board of Health and Welfare are involved in the central steering of public health care. These include the Board for Social Insurance, the Labour Protection Board, the National Laboratory of Bacteriology, the Board for the Further Education of Physicians, the Sanitary Board, the Responsibility Board and the Board for the Expansion of the Teaching Hospitals. Two central agencies that are semi-private in nature – Landstingsförbundet and SPRI – enter this coordination and negotiation system. These two bodies play a major role in creating national norms for the structuring of the health care system. They operate by means of investigations, recommendations and advice, but their points of view are often very authoritative. This applies in particular to the Federation, which not only participates in a number of commissions and boards but also negotiates materially with both the government and the trade unions.

What are the implications for the health care professionals of this major organizational transition, from a state-centred model to a decentralized model underlining the planning role of the county councils? Health professionals attempt to maintain autonomy at hospitals and other health care institutions. How is this autonomy affected by decentralization? Also, in a public system of health care, professionals strive to attain influence over crucial policy-making in order to protect their interests. How is this influence affected by the decentralization of power to the local government tier?

Professionals and Public Policy-Making: Influence

The Swedish health system has been changed completely in volume, organization and goals. These changes have transformed the role of the professionals. In the old system most physicians were partly salaried by their public employer, partly paid fees for services. The health consumer, on the other hand, had to pay a large part of the costs from his/her own pocket. Today over 90 percent of physicians are publicly employed, and the health consumers pay only a small fixed sum; almost all health costs are financed by taxes and public insurances. By the introduction of salaried public employment, the physicians lost part of their special status. These changes in the health system were introduced by central political decisions. The following may be mentioned as milestones (Bjurulf and Swahn 1980):

1 In 1928 the county councils were obliged to arrange hospital care.
2 In 1959 the county councils were instructed to arrange ambulatory care in the hospitals.
3 In 1961 the county councils were obliged to arrange out-patient clinics outside the hospitals.
4 In 1970 the seven crowns reform was introduced, which fixed the consumer rate for an ambulatory or out-patient care visit.
5 In 1972 guidelines for decentralization of specialists from hospital care to out-patient care were introduced.
6 In 1982 the new Health and Sick Care Law (the HSL) was introduced, which gave the county councils more power over health care delivery.

The main cleavage in health politics has been between the Social Democratic Party and the Swedish Medical Association. However, it should be emphasized that most decisions concerning health care have been taken with political unanimity. Antagonism between the ruling Social Democratic Party and the SMA characterized health care policy-making until the 1960s. The SMA in general opposed various proposals, but never managed to change the direction of the health policy. At the beginning of the 1970s, clashes between the government and the SMA became less frequent, which reflected changes in the cadre of the SMA. A new generation of physicians had been educated to work in a public health system, and therefore had a perspective close to that of the government. By the end of the

1970s the interaction between the SMA and the political system again became antagonistic, because of the introduction of the new Health Law (Serner 1980; Heidenheimer 1980).

The 1982 legislation: from bill to law
Most health professional interest groups to which the HSL bill was submitted for consideration were negative about the proposal. In general, these bodies argued that the HSL was too vague and lacked substance. They also opposed abolition of the detailed rules in the 1962 law as well as the potential lack of central control. The SMA maintained that quality, security and effectiveness could not be guaranteed without detailed rules, emphasizing professional competence.

The Federation of Swedish County Councils and the county councils themselves were on the whole positive about the HSL, and found its overall framework attractive. The HSL would provide them with the right to make decisions about the content and organization of health care, which would make it possible for public representatives to adapt health care to the needs of a particular county. Because of the extended definition of health care in the HSL compared with the law of 1962, new categories of professionals (such as social welfare workers) appreciated the HSL. A balanced position was held by the SHSTF, which organizes among others nurses, midwives and ward sisters. It argued that the HSL was somewhat vague, but agreed to the basic framework (Proposition 1981/82: 97).

The positions for or against the HSL bill involved two cleavages. The first consisted of the county councils and the Federation of County Councils versus the organizations of the health professionals, mainly the SMA. The second consisted of trade unions which organized the less educated health workers and the administrators versus the health professionals, again mainly the SMA. These cleavages centre on a tangible and controversial clause in the HSL proposal: the abolition of the detailed rules in the 1962 law that regulate the structure of health care organization and the responsibilities of professionals.

The law of 1962 stated that the head of the clinic should be a physician. Furthermore, it regulated in detail the responsibilities of the personnel in certain positions. Among other things it was stated that the ultimate medical responsibility rested with an appointed physician. The HSL bill proposed that no regulation of the responsibilities of various personnel was needed. Moreover, no regulation of administrative responsibility or organizational rules was needed. These were instead to be regulated by the county council itself. Finally, the medical responsibility of physicians was to be retained at different levels. One consequence of this proposal was that the head of a clinic need no longer be a physician, because of the separation of administrative and medical responsibility. Another consequence was that medical responsibility would no longer rest with a particular physician.

Almost all county councils and the Federation of County Councils agreed with the proposal. To Federation it was evident that the county councils themselves could choose the structure of the organization that suited them best. However, this freedom did not prevent the existing organization from being retained, if such suited a county council.

The organizations of health professionals were negative or hesitant. The SHSTF opposed the provision that political representatives should decide if certain skills were needed for superior positions. The SMA argued that it was impossible to separate administrative and medical responsibilities. The SMA maintained that the head of the clinic or the block should still be a physician, and that medical responsibility should rest with an appointed physician. Other trade unions argued that if medical responsibility were to be regulated by law, then it should also include other professional categories. The SSR which organizes social welfare workers found reasons to abolish medical responsibility completely by arguing that various kinds of professionals must have equal status.

The HSL bill passed through parliament without any major changes. At one point criticism resulted in changes in the final law: the ultimate medical responsibility could rest with an appointed physician, but the National Board of Health and Welfare could allow the exercise of health care by a person without medical responsibility. In terms of gains and losses, the county councils and the Federation were the winners. The HSL increased county council control over the organization and the sphere of health care. The extension of the health concept opened up opportunities for other categories to increase their influence. The losers were the traditional health professionals.

Professional Power in a Decentralized System: Autonomy

Health care provision in the Swedish system is a fusion of political and medical organizations, integrated into a politico-administrative system. Owing to regional variation, it is not possible to describe the health care organization by a general model applicable to all county councils. However, the structure of the health organization may be outlined in a simplified model (Figure 3.1).

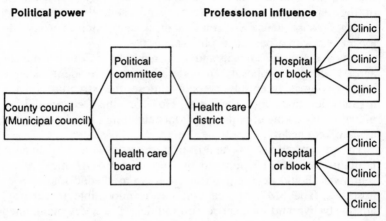

Figure 3.1   *Regional and local structure of the health care organization in Sweden*

In this model, political power rests with the county council, which consists of elected public representatives. The county council decides budgets, taxes, and overall organization as well as dimensioning of health care. To implement decisions, prepare items for the agenda and maintain ongoing operations, each county has a committee (*förvaltningsutskott*) partly consisting of full-time politicians. There is also a health care board that has overall responsibility for planning health care in the county council (in some county councils the *förvaltningsutskott* also acts as the health care board). The law requires a unit in the organization of the county council with such an overall function. While this unit has been described in detail in the health care law of 1962, the law of 1982 gives the county councils more discretion to choose their particular form of organization.

The health organization is divided by geographical or medical criteria into the smaller units of the health care districts and hospital administrations. In general, the districts comprise various hospitals, units for out-patient care and so on, which are brought together under the same political and administrative direction. This is – with some exceptions – the lowest level at which politicians act in the organization. The health care districts are linked to the operative units by the hospital director, who generally is an administrator. The director coordinates and exercises administrative responsibility for the aggregated health care units, which might consist of a block of clinics. The blocks are groups of clinics with similar medical specialties.

In addition to the hospital director there is a chief physician, who is responsible for medical coordination. From here and downwards in the organization, administrative responsibility is combined with medical responsibility. In the law of 1962 both of these responsibilities rested with physicians. This changed in the law of 1982.

It is obvious that the politicians have the power over organization and economy, while the professionals take responsibility for delivery of health care. The politicians may affect the care in the professional sphere by decisions concerning organization and budgets, which define the boundaries for the health professionals. The politicians also decide on investments in medical technology. The health professionals act in the political sphere only as consultants. In general, physicians for in-patient and out-patient care participate as experts on medical issues.

Another way for professionals to have an impact is to engage in negotiations according to the MBL scheme, the codetermination law of 1976. To the health care organization, the consequence of the MBL is that no changes can take place before negotiations between the trade unions and the employer.

The interaction among politicians and health professionals at local level is shaped by the laws and activities enacted and directed by the central government. The relation between the political sphere and the professional sphere was clearly defined in the health care law of 1962. The HSL differs from the former law in three ways: the basic concept has been extended from sick care to health and sick care; the detailed rules of various kinds of responsibilities and relations have been abolished and replaced by general goals and a vaguely defined framework; and, as a consequence of the abolition of the detailed rules plus the ambition to decentralize power over health care, central government power has diminished.

The HSL law does not contain any new programme to be implemented, or any new goal to be fulfilled. It extends county council discretion over the organization and content of health care. The extension of the health concept has caused concern over what it implies. Today the county councils partly translate the new health concept into preventive health care, and organizations with this function are expanding.

However, to date, there have been few major changes in the health care system. The power to give administrative responsibility to categories other than physicians has seldom been used. There are very few clinics where the administrative responsibility rests with other kinds of personnel (such as a physiotherapy clinic where the responsibility rests with a physiotherapist). In general the county councils have retained the organization that existed before the HSL, which means that administrative responsibility rests with a physician. The HSL admitted the opportunity to carry on health care without personnel with medical responsibility under certain conditions and after an application to the National Board of Health and Welfare. By 1985 only a couple of such applications had been received by the Board; neither had been accepted.

The power of the politicians in the county council has been increased by the HSL, but it could be argued that they have a limited space for changing decisions. The economic predicament limits the ability to initiate new programmes; decisions mainly concern the maintenance of or a change in the priorities of existing programmes. To increase efficiency there are tendencies towards the decentralization of decisions and economic responsibility. In some county councils this has resulted in a reorganization providing greater influence and responsibility for the physicians at the clinical level. The newly introduced budget system, the so-called 'base unit system', places economic responsibility with the head of the clinic. This generally allows a higher degree of freedom for the clinic head to decide about resources. Because of decentralization and the new budget system, the autonomy of the health professionals seems to be retained if not increased at the clinical level. Even though the HSL opened up the possibility for county councils to change the health organization fundamentally, this has not occurred. The health system is complex and has great inertia, and changes have to be negotiated according to the MBL.

Public Health Care Systems: Politics and Technology

A public health care system involves a number of organizations and clients. Given the many demands to be recognized, it seems very difficult to derive any simple solution to the structuring of the system. Consider the Swedish health care system on a unit level. The system consists of a large number of hospitals organized in terms of the county council system. The hospital system involves three layers: 8 regional hospitals, 26 county hospitals, 89 community hospitals and 19 mental hospitals as well as 247 long-term treatment institutions. The number of private hospital institutions is 207, but these units are typically very small ones engaged in long-term treatment. There is also a rapidly developing system of community health clinics constituting so-called primary care. Who is to decide about the size and orientation of these units?

Centralization versus decentralization

If health care were only a matter for a regional group of citizens, then everything could be left with the county councils. However, this is not the case. The provision of health care concerns more people than those who happen to live in a certain area at a particular time. The citizens may find it difficult to accept that moving to a new county could mean a very different kind of health care. Thus there is a demand for standardization. Moreover, an externality also is involved because it is in the interest of all citizens that people in various areas are provided with similar basic health care. The emphasis on equality becomes even stronger when one considers the costs of regional health care. However strong the demand for regionalization of health care services may be, it is not considered acceptable that citizens in various regions pay differently for such a fundamental welfare service according to the circumstances that happen to pertain in a single region or county. Thus, there is a drive for state grants and state supervision of the quantity and quality of health care.

The strong national goods characteristic of health care is at odds with the heavy organizational emphasis upon the regional principals, the county councils. The inherent conflict between the types of goods involved and the prevailing organizational structure becomes even more pronounced when one considers the logic of health care technology. The interpretation of health care as a national or a local public good is not stationary but rather affected by the evolution of health care technologies. It is no exaggeration to claim that health care develops in a way that makes it less dependent on local resources. Since it becomes possible to treat more and more patients with ever more advanced technologies in shorter times, the local supply of health care may involve serious inefficiencies. Local or regional provision of health may fail to reap considerable scale economies. This works in two ways.

An allocation of health care resources in terms of a national perspective will mean that it may prove advantageous from a technological point of view to concentrate some resources at certain places in order to make the specialization of health care economically feasible. This process works both within regions and between regions. It is no longer economically defensible to commit large amounts of resources to community hospitals when there is rapid access to both county hospitals and regional hospitals. In fact, the needs of the patient may imply that it is not appropriate to treat certain types of diseases at community hospitals or even county hospitals when advanced treatment is available at a regional hospital. However, it is far from obvious that the organizational structure emphasizing decentralization is accessible to such region-wide considerations. This is even more acute when it becomes necessary to plan the health resources in such a way that some resources have to be concentrated at a special regional hospital. How is this kind of nation-wide coordination to become a possibility when the power of the centre is weakened in terms of an extensive decentralization process?

Not only may intercounty concentration be hampered by the process of decentralization, but also intracounty concentration will likely meet strong resistance in a decentralized system. There will simply be too many other kinds of circumstances for the county council to take into account when allocating health care resources besides health care technology and economy. In county council decision-making it has until now been the case that the major organizational units – the big hospitals – have proved strong enough to resist major structural innovations stemming from the need for new forms of health care. The traditional hospital-based structure may resist the requirements for change owing to considerations of between-county as well as within-county coordination. Thus, organizational structure as well as organizational interests may work against technological and economic imperatives.

The position of the professionals
It may be believed that decentralization always furthers the interests of health professionals, because the power or discretion allocated from the centre to the local level automatically ends up with the professionals. This is hardly the case. It depends on how the professionals fit into the existing structure at local level.

Swedish health professionals have by tradition had three ways to improve their situation. One alternative has diminished: this was to become a private practitioner with one's own clinic. Although there were some spectacular attempts to revive private health care in the early 1980s, the private alternative in the control of the provision of health care is not going to be an option for many professionals.

The second alternative is to possess a large degree of autonomy within a public system for health provision, whether state centred or local government oriented. Swedish health professionals have had to cope with both organizational directives about the structuring of institutions and rules of conduct for the protection of patients. These directives were previously state initiated to a large extent, but the process of decentralization has definitely increased the role of county councils and the three municipalities outside the county council system. Although health professionals have substantial amounts of autonomy in organizing and directing the provision of care within various clinics and institutions, the overall system of policy-making has not been entrusted to them. While the state once planned the organizational development of the health care system, now local governments are much more involved. Moreover, outside control of health care remains as the *ex post facto* review process involves a real threat of punishment against malpractice.

The third alternative is to influence external decision-making that limits the autonomy of professionals. Representative health professionals have tried to take an active role in shaping both organizational decision-making and the conduct of health care. Thus, professionals participate at both central and local level in order to influence various kinds of decisions (Björkman 1985a). They have a role in planning bodies as well as in peer review bodies at the centre. Moreover, they negotiate with local government politicians and planners about structuring hospitals and institutions.

The crucial problem is whether the combination of autonomy and influence which delimits health professionals will be positively affected by the decentralization process. Our argument is that this is questionable. It may prove more difficult to protect professional discretion and maintain influence in a decentralized system for the reasons outlined above. Local government considerations may outweigh professional interests, which are centred on the technology of health care rather than on the local organizational demands of the county councils.

Conclusion

The performance of health care systems is crucially dependent on the motivation and competence of health professionals. The provision of health care is looked upon as a public function in Sweden, and the problem is one of how to integrate health professionals into a political structure. Health professionals may control the provision of health care either by autonomy from politicians and administrators or by influence over the decisions of politicians and administrators. In Sweden we find both mechanisms at work. At the same time as the private sector for health care services has been almost abolished, health professionals have maintained some degree of freedom at the basic units – the clinics – while they have participated in various national government decision processes that have affected the basic units.

The most pervasive change in the Swedish health care system relates to the introduction in 1982 of far-reaching decentralization which emphasized the role of the local government system at the expense of the national government. The decentralization process could constitute a threat to the position of health professionals, in particular physicians, as politicians and administrators at regional level have much greater control over the health care system. Regional planning will replace central planning to a considerable extent. And the position of the health professionals will be dependent on their capacity to participate in regional decision-making processes where politicians and administrators constitute a strong group. It is far from obvious that decentralization means more power for health professionals. It may even be argued that decentralization reflects political circumstances rather than the technological and economic requirements of health care provision. Health care is hardly a pure type of local good.

4

Controlling Dutch Health Care

*Nico Baakman, Jan van der Made
and Ingrid Mur-Veeman*

The Dutch health care system presents a unique case. It strikingly displays a basic feature of the Dutch political system, which, in line with the work of Lijphart (1968) and the debate on neo-corporatism, can best be labelled 'consociational corporatism'. In other words, although health care is largely a public affair, for historical reasons the government controls it only in a rather limited sense (Schrijvers and Boot 1983).

In the years between 1813 (when the present Dutch state was founded) and 1945 the government abstained from entering the health sector, so private organizations conquered the field. When some form of state action became unavoidable, the government found itself confronted with well-established organizations which claimed jurisdiction over health care. When the state intervened it made no attempt to annex or incorporate them but rather tried to accommodate them. One intervention – and a decisive one – was the enactment of the medical statute in 1865 which provided uniform rules for professional training, a legal monopoly to academically trained physicians, severe penalties on unqualified practitioners, and a state inspection of health care (Cannegieter 1954). The statute was promoted by the Royal Dutch Society for the Advancement of Medicine (KNMG), itself founded for this purpose in 1849 (Festen 1974). KNMG still exists, and its two formally independent branches of specialists and general practitioners (GPs) are very influential.

Health care ranks prominently among the functions of the welfare state. In recent years its share of GNP has reached 10 percent, about three-quarters of which is public money. When economic crisis and a change in political climate required financial austerity, and therefore more control over health care, the latter proved to be no easy target. Control over health care involves dominance over three related areas of decisions: prices; medical consumption or volume (what facilities, where and how many); and the financial system (who pays for what and in what way). The Dutch government has tried to structure its system along these lines, especially since 1974 when Parliament unanimously accepted an important government paper as the basis for future policy.

From 1945 to 1974

The war did great damage to the Dutch economy, and the first post-war election brought Christian and Social Democrats together in the cabinet. Their main target was to keep the costs of labour down in order to stimulate investment and economic growth. In the field of health care this was done in a number of ways. Hospital tariffs were under strict control as were all prices. Because of the scarcity of building materials, there was an annual budget for the (re)construction of hospitals, and sickness fund premiums were set at the lowest possible level. Charges by GPs were fixed, and central government gave as little subsidy to the Cross Societies (principal actors in public health care in the Netherlands) as was politically possible (Juffermans 1982). Macro-economically the government set the rules of the game very strictly, but it failed to plan the structure of the health system.

During the post-war years an important change took place in Dutch health care. The hospital changed from a place to nurse the sick into a therapeutic institution. Before the war, the bulk of health care was delivered by GPs. After it, hospitals and specialists took over. They did so for technical reasons, but also because after a German decree of 1941 the sickness funds paid for hospital care. This development caused an escalation of costs and a steady growth in the number of specialists.

Again private initiative took the lead by using public money. In 1950 only 37 of the 250 hospitals belonged to the state, whereas 112 were run by Roman Catholics, 43 by Protestants, and 58 by secular organizations. Between 1940 and 1960 the number of available hospital beds rose from 32,000 to 58,000 (Juffermans 1982). Existing hospitals were enlarged and new ones built at places where private organizations thought it proper, rather than where they might be most needed. Building continued until the annual budget was spent and sometimes beyond, with no regard for national priorities – largely because the central government provided none. After the budget was spent, the next applicant in principle had to wait until the following year. This kind of 'planning' created a very odd distribution of facilities, a fact which did not go unnoticed. In 1949 minister Joekes (Social Democrat) tried to get a planning bill enacted, but he failed because of strong opposition from the confessional parties – mainly the Catholics – who had and have close ties with the well-established private organizations.

These organizations often competed with each other on the local level. Muntendam (1983), once the highest civil servant of the health department, has presented a nice example. A small town in a Protestant region had a well-functioning Roman Catholic hospital. It had been there for decades; it recruited both staff and patients from the region, and so many of both were Protestants. The mayors of the surrounding municipalities, however, supported by the local churches, wanted a wholly Protestant and therefore a second hospital. To everybody involved it was clear that, should they succeed, one hospital would necessarily fail. It proved impossible to convince the zealots that such a project would waste public money and, since Muntendam had no legal means to stop them, they had to be bought off. They got a Protestant hospital for the chronically ill. It prevented the bankruptcy of one institution, but did little to stimulate balanced development of the health system. Private, that is confessional, organizations had become powerful, not least because they had strong backing in Parliament where many MPs also held positions in the same organizations.

Public health care had become the virtual monopoly of the Cross Societies, but these had become dependent on government subsidies. The subsidy was based upon their battle against tuberculosis, although they performed many other tasks as well. Therefore they wanted it increased, something they obtained in 1952. The Cross Societies were pleased, of course, but not at all satisfied. They preferred a reliable flow of money from the government rather than an uncertain subsidy which was decided anew each year. A subsidy law would have suited their wishes, or alternatively money could have been provided through the social insurance system. Eventually the latter happened, but only in the late 1970s.

In 1949 the Sickness Fund Council was established as the official cabinet advisory board on all sickness fund matters including the premium rates. The premium is a percentage of the wage below an upper limit, of which half is paid by the employer and half by the employee. Since there was strict price control, the Social Economic Council (SER) also advised the minister on all prices. Often it advised a lower premium rate than did the Sickness Fund Council, because it wanted to keep the costs of labour down. The cabinet always followed the SER's advice (Juffermans 1982). The same policy was adopted with regard to the hospital tariffs; these were set as low as possible, thus forcing the hospitals (and the sickness funds) to use up their accumulated savings. This financial squeeze was only acceptable because price control was generally considered to be one of the major pillars of reconstruction. It could not, however, last indefinitely.

In 1950, the scientific staff bureau of the Catholic Party produced a report on health care. The Christian Democrats objected to government interference in health care, although it did not really go far beyond price control. Yet the private initiative organizations wanted exclusive jurisdiction wherein government would provide only the money. The 1950 report has been the foundation for Dutch health politics for many years.

In 1956 the Central Health Council was set up. A typical example of the post-war cooperation of the private organizations and the government, it institutionalized consultation among the relevant interest groups, but made no attempt to restructure the health field. The Council advised the government – and its advice was almost always followed because of its strong backing by the confessional parties in Parliament, notwithstanding the fact that the organizations represented on the Council were often competing with each other at the local level. In Amsterdam, indeed, they competed not only with each other but also with local government institutions. One must bear in mind that the city ran several hospitals and was the first to establish a municipal health service (Verdoorn 1981).

In December 1958 there was a split in the coalition between Social Democrats and Catholics which had ruled the country since the end of the war. As the years of reconstruction were over, the Christian Democrats no longer needed the Socialists; the former took over, supported by the Liberals (in the Netherlands really conservatives, although less so in the first post-war years). That meant the end of the modest government control that existed at the time. The building and the tariffs of hospitals were 'liberated', so that if funds could be raised – and they easily could, for no health institution in the Netherlands ever went bankrupt – a local government automatically issued a building permit. Nothing could stop the construction of hospital facilities. Tariffs were negotiated between the sickness funds and the hospital organizations, the former always being the weaker party. Because the law guaranteed the insured medical care and not reimbursement of costs, the hospitals could always corner the sickness funds, for the latter had to implement the law.

Perpetual quarrels characterized the field until finally the minister made the two parties understand that if they would not develop stable forms of cooperation he would impose them. The parties responded, and in 1965 the Hospital Tariffs Act was enacted (de Wolff 1984). While it provided some control over tariffs, none of these dealt with medical consumption, which soon became the real problem. As a consequence of the law, the Central Organization for Hospital Tariffs (COZ) was established, composed of the sickness funds and the hospital organizations which jointly set the tariffs. While the minister could overrule its decisions with regard to the national economic situation, he never did. COZ ruled supreme, although it was a *stichting*, that is a private law body. The years after 1965 witnessed a slow but steady growth of its tasks. Although functioning on a very weak legal basis, it determined more and more prices in health care (de Wolff 1984).

Yet the costs did not go down. In 1966 the Sickness Funds Insurance Act replaced the 1941 decree, but the new law merely codified the existing situation. In that same year the government produced a health care report which described the state of affairs but made no political choices. Nothing changed. Organizations in the field made use of every opportunity for growth, without any thoughts about a structure or a national plan.

In 1967 Parliament passed the General Special Sickness Expenses Act. It supplemented the Sickness Fund Insurance Act by covering heavy risks, like prolonged treatment, for the whole population. Implemented by the sickness funds and the commercial insurance companies, its premiums are paid by employers as a percentage of the wage. Since January 1980 most of the costs of the Cross Societies have also been met this way – partly to camouflage health costs, because subsidies appear on the budget whereas social insurance premiums do not. Yet the Dutch could not delude themselves indefinitely.

The first serious attempt to structure the field was made in 1971 through the Hospital Facilities Act. The law was only to come into force after the drafting of a national hospital plan, and it forbade the building of a hospital not included in the plan. The planning procedure, however, was made so complicated (because every organization in the field had to have a say in it) that no national plan was ever established. The law came into force in 1979, but the Act is still not very effective.

By 1974 it had become clear to everyone that the time had come to stop the growth of health care costs, be it only for macroeconomic reasons. The then Secretary of State published a new Memorandum on the Structure of the Health Services, which Parliament approved unanimously. This Memorandum argued the need for more government intervention and promised to enlarge the influence of local and regional governments. It also emphasized primary care in order to reduce dependence on expensive hospitals, and recommended more preventive and non-residential care (that is more care by GPs and Cross Societies). The overall number of hospital beds was to be reduced, the Hospital Tariffs Act was to be expanded to cover all health care prices, and a Health Services Act would replace the Hospital Facilities Act. This agenda was nothing less than a potential revolution. In the face of great difficulties, audacity may well have been needed. But making ambitious plans is one thing; implementing them is quite another.

The Mini-Revolution of 1974 and What Came of It

The developments leading to the Memorandum of 1974 were: a minimum of government interference; a complicated and differentiated financial system; an unbalanced growth leading to excessive emphasis on in-patient care and too little on ambulatory and preventive care; a lack of internal functional coherence; and the mushrooming of organizations (commonly called quangos) around the state bureaucracy which perform public tasks and dominate decision-making at the national level (Johnson 1979). Quangos are very important and are frequently used in Dutch health care. The most important ones for supply, cost, and the financing system are the Council of Hospital Facilities, the National Health Council, the Central Organization for Health Tariffs and the Sickness Fund Council. The National Health Council and the Council of Hospital Facilities are purely advisory bodies. Most members of these four quangos are representatives of interest groups or local authorities. In addition some members are appointed for their expertise, but civil servants in the Department of Health are excluded from membership. They may, however, attend as non-voting advisers (Hofland and Wilms 1984).

The remarkable nature of the 1974 Memorandum on the Structure of the Health Services cannot be overexaggerated. It announced no less than the restructuring of the health field through more government influence. More specifically it envisioned cost control through measures regarding price and financing, and enlarged controllability through matching supply and demand. These plans had to be executed along five lines: regionalization, echeloning, administrative organization, democratization, and legislation.

The Memorandum became the starting point for a wave of new laws and measures, which created new patterns of decisional power in Dutch health care. These can be grouped as mechanisms regarding control of supply, price and cost regulation, and regulation of financing (Rutten and Van der Werff 1982). The control of supply was directed to control of quantity, structure and quality of the available facilities. It came under two Acts: the Hospital Facilities Act and the Health Services Act.

Supply control

The most important ministerial powers or instruments in the Hospital Facilities Act concern the planning of hospital capacity, the issuing of building permits and the closure of hospitals. At the minister's request, the provinces must prepare regional hospital plans which specify the types of facilities (hospitals, nursing homes, and so on), the region(s) to be covered, and the financial limits. Each plan specifies the capacity and functions of facilities, states their optimal future level and indicates the way(s) to achieve it.

In order to guarantee the participation of the different parties concerned, the provinces must follow certain procedures which lead to a proposal drawn up by the provincial council. This is sent to the minister and to the Council of Hospital Facilities. The task of the latter quango is to advise the minister on the implementation of the Hospital Facilities Act. It consists of 25 members of whom the chairman is appointed by the government as a whole and the other members by the minister. Apart from two independent members the Council has representatives from organizations of hospitals, medical professions, financing bodies (sickness funds and private health insurance companies), municipalities, provinces, employers and employees. The seats are distributed as shown in Table 4.1. It is striking that the organizations of hospital facilities and medical professionals occupy nearly half the seats. Moreover, since medical professionals are amply represented in the organizations of financing bodies, the suppliers clearly dominate decision-making. The influence of employers and employees is minimal, while consumers occupy only one seat.

After the advice of the Council of Hospital Facilities, the minister finalizes the plan. If his version contains alterations of the proposal, the parties concerned may appeal to the government. Its approval will render the plan definitive and valid for a period of four years. No province has a free hand when drawing up its proposal. The ministerial directives serve as guidelines, and therefore as the basis for the final plan. These directives are manifold and highly detailed; they concern the structure of the plan (prospects, aims, and so on) and specific types of facilities.

The next important instrument is the permit. The law says that the construction of new hospitals and the extension, renovation, replacement, and alteration of existing ones are subject to ministerial approval.

If a particular hospital facility does not fit the official plan, the minister may decide to close down all or parts of it. The same may be done if it is no longer accredited by the Sickness Fund Insurance Act or the General Special Sickness Expenses Act. Before taking a

Table 4.1 *Distribution of seats in Dutch health care quangos (1987 figures)*

	Council of Hospital Facilities		National Health Council[1]		Central Organization for Health Tariffs		Sickness Fund Council	
	Number	Percent	Number	Percent	Number	Percent	Number	Percent
Health care institutions and medical professionals	12	48	30	67	4	22	9	23
Financing bodies	5	20	4	9	4	22	9	23
Provinces and municipalities	3	12	4	9	–	–	–	–
Employers	1	4	2	4	2	11	7	18
Employees	1	4	2	4	2	11	7	18
Consumers	1	4	3	7	–	–	–	–
Independent experts	2	8	–	–	6	34	7	18
Total seats	25	100	45	100	18	100	39	100

[1]On the National Health Council the votes differ from the seats: see text.

decision of this kind the minister must consult the Council of Hospital Facilities and the provincial council involved, and the latter must consult the hospital and local authorities concerned.

By the end of 1988 the minister had ordered 102 proposals to be drawn up by the provincial councils. Actually 24 proposals have been drawn up and 17 plans have been finalized. This should not lead one to conclude that the provinces have done very little. Based on a section in the Act dealing with the closure of hospitals and prompted by the minister, most of the provinces have submitted proposals for a reduction of the number of hospital beds.

The Health Services Act seeks to control the supply of almost all health facilities in order to achieve decentralization, democratization and cohesion in the whole health services system. Its aim is very broad and reaches beyond mere volume control. At present, however, although passed by Parliament in 1982, the Health Services Act is not fully in force and probably never will be. As a result of a change in the political climate, people are less in favour of planning and more in favour of deregulation. Whether or not the Act will be withdrawn is uncertain. The most important instruments of the Act are planning and accreditation, establishment and size of practice, and prescription of quality standards.

Under the Health Services Act planning would also be done by municipalities. In principle they would be responsible for planning primary care facilities through a procedure much like that under the Hospital Facilities Act. The provincial plan would need governmental approval, and the municipal one had to be approved of by the provincial executives. The National Health Council advises the minister on the Health Services Act. Advice on the Health Services Act is not the only task of the National Health Council, for it also advises on structure, implementation, quality, legislation, efficiency, and indeed on all matters concerning health care.

In addition, the Council attempts to promote cooperation among the authorities and private organizations in the field. It has 45 members, with its seats distributed as shown in Table 4.1. However, the number of votes differs from the number of seats. The votes of the representatives of the financing bodies, provinces, municipalities, employers, employees and consumers count double so, taken together, their votes match those of the suppliers of health care. Nevertheless, since medical professionals are also represented on the financing bodies, the suppliers of health care have the greatest influence on the National Health Council.

Health care services offered by independent medical professionals are not covered by the planning procedure of the Health Services Act. Volume control in this area is achieved by separate regulations in the law concerning location and size of practice. The law can dictate that a specific category of (medical) professionals is not allowed to set up practice in (part of) the country without a permit. So far this only applies to GPs. At present this regulation is one of the few parts of the law which are in force.

Price and cost control

The second line of regulatory mechanisms concerns price and cost control, based particularly on the Health Tariffs Act, various budgetary measures, and the Financial Survey of Health Care. The Health Tariffs Act was implemented in 1982 and replaces the Hospital Tariffs Act of 1965 which only allowed price control of in-patient health care. The more extensive Health Tariffs Act applies to the entire field of health care. The act rules that all tariffs and fees need the approval of the Central Organization for Health Tariffs. Tariffs are fixed according to the following procedure. In principle the organizations of medical professionals and institutions first meet the organizations of financing bodies to discuss tariffs. If they agree, the tariff will be submitted for approval to the Central Organization. If they cannot reach an agreement, the Central Organization may officially or by request establish the tariff. If they wish, the parties concerned may express their views.

The Central Organization then examines the tariff on the basis of directives as to the size, structure and calculation of the tariff. The directives are, as it were, the limits within which the parties are free to bargain. They are established by the Central Organization itself, independently or on ministerial guidelines from the Minister of Health and/or the Minister of Economic Affairs. These directives require ratification by the minister. Decisions on tariffs taken by the Central Organization may be suspended or nullified by government at a later stage on grounds of their being against the law or not in the public interest. In addition, anyone whose interest is harmed by a decision on tariffs may appeal to the Professional Appeals Board.

The Central Organization for Health Tariffs plays an important role in the process of price regulation. It not only approves tariffs, but also develops directives, and advises the government on all subjects concerning price development in health care. The Central Organization consists of eighteen members of whom six are appointed by the government, four by the minister after consultation with the organizations of the health care institutions and medical professionals, another four after consultation with the organizations of financing bodies, and the final four after consultation with the organizations of employers and employees (Table 4.1).

The law requires that the members of the Central Organization must not be professionally involved with the organizations of health institutions, professionals, and financing bodies which participate in the discussions on tariffs. They can be members of these organizations, though nomination by the various interest organizations is not binding; members of the Central Organization are appointed after consultation.

There are six subcommittees for various categories of health care institutions which come under the Central Organization. The members of these committees are representatives of the organizations of health care institutions, medical professionals, and financing bodies. The seats of the first two together equal those of the third. Members of the committees need not be members of the Central Organization itself; they are nominated by the afore-mentioned organizations and appointed by the Central Organization. The only task of these committees is to advise on directives. They are not involved in the establishment of tariffs. Although the members of the Central Organization do not directly represent the interest organizations which recommended them for membership to the minister, they belong to them and are likely to consider the interests of their organizations. They are thus interested parties when decisions are taken.

Significantly, consumer organizations again are not represented. However, the suppliers of health care have considerably fewer seats (proportionally) than on other bodies, and independent experts play a more important role. The influence of suppliers and financing bodies is limited, and that of consumers nil. On the other hand the committees, whose role in the development of directives is important, allow the suppliers and financing bodies to have much greater influence. Here, they control half of the total number of seats.

In 1983, hospitals had to abandon the tariff system in favour of the system of budget financing because hospital costs account for an enormous share of total health care costs. From 1984 budget financing has also been applied to all other in-patient health services. The term 'budget financing' stands for a system by which institutions receive a budget in advance from which to finance the health care services. It is important that costs do not exceed the limits, in order not to jeopardize future budgets. Budgets are fixed by the Central Organization for Health Tariffs after consultation with health institutions and financing bodies. However, since the system does not cover the services of medical specialists, budget financing cannot achieve total control of in-patient health care costs.

Finally, the annual *Financial Survey of Health Care* (published by the government since 1977) not only contains an analysis of costs made in the entire health care system, but also gives a forecast of costs for three years ahead. This framework functions as a target for the government and an indicator for the social insurance institutions.

Finance control

Control of financing (the third regulatory mechanism) is based primarily on the social insurance schemes of the Sickness Fund Insurance Act and the General Special Sickness Expenses Act. The Sickness Fund Insurance Act gives those insured (61 percent of the total population) the right to medical care, such as basic and specialist treatment, obstetric, hospital and psychiatric treatment, and so on. The nature, content and amount of medical care is described in a decree which accompanies the Act, the so-called coverage decree. Implementation of the Act rests with the sickness funds, which stipulate contracts with organizations and individuals providing health care. Those insured with one of the 52 sickness funds have to approach an institution or (medical) professional who has a contract with that particular sickness fund. Negotiations about the contents of contracts take place between the sickness funds and the organizations of health care institutions and professionals. When agreement has been reached, the contract (except the part dealing with the tariffs) is submitted to the Sickness Fund Council for approval. In addition, the Sickness Fund Council advises the government and the Ministers of Health and Social Affairs on all matters concerning the Sickness Fund Insurance Act and the General Special Sickness Expenses Act.

The Sickness Fund Council has 39 members, appointed by the organizations of employers, employees, sickness funds, private health insurance companies, health care institutions and medical professionals. In addition a number of independent experts are appointed by the minister. The distribution of the seats is shown in Table 4.1.

The minister may advise the Council on the performance of its task. Decisions taken by the Council, if incompatible with the law or the public interest, may be suspended or nullified by government. Interested parties may appeal to government against a number of Council decisions (such as those on payments to executive bodies).

The distribution of representatives in the Council indicates that employers and employees have more influence than they have in other quangos. The number of their seats almost equals that of the other interest groups; we may therefore conclude that there is a fair representation of interests. The only group not represented is that of consumer organizations.

As the General Special Sickness Expenses Act (1967) deals with the insurance of all residents of the Netherlands against exceptional medical expenses, it applies to facilities and services such as nursing and treatment in hospitals and psychiatric and mental institutions for longer than 365 days. Implementation of the Act rests with the sickness funds, private health insurance companies and executive bodies of civil servants' health insurance schemes. The Sickness Fund Insurance Act and the General Special Sickness Expenses Act state that every institution which offers health care and requires financing from the funds of these Acts must have ministerial accreditation. The minister grants accreditation mainly on the basis of quality criteria. Prior to taking a decision on accreditation the minister will ask the advice of the Sickness Fund Council.

Discussion and Conclusion

This chapter has described the Dutch health services system from 1945 to the present. This period has been divided into two – before and after 1974. For many years, until the end of World War II, health care ranked low among the priorities of the Dutch government. Government abstained as much as it could, leaving the field to societal initiative. Many organizations were established, and they made full use of the growth possibilities of the welfare state between 1945 and 1974. In that period government restricted itself to safeguarding these organizations and their income. But this situation led to an unbalanced expansion and an explosion of costs. The Dutch health care system was characterized by a minimum of government interference, a complex financial system, a lack of internal coherence, and many predominantly para-governmental organizations. Parliamentary acceptance of the ministerial Memorandum on the Structure of Health Care in 1974 marks the end of this period, after which a phase of attempted governmental control began.

How successful were those attempts? It is obvious that government interference increased, while the autonomy of health care facilities and professionals decreased. A recent study (Honigh 1985) points out that government does make use of its new powers, especially where the building of new hospitals is concerned. But the Council of Hospital Facilities quango (with its strong representation from hospital facilities and professionals) seems to be very influential because of its leading role in communications about these measures. Also most advice from the Council was accepted by the ministry and seemed to outweigh the provincial advice. Hitherto the role of the provinces and municipalities in health policy-making has been limited. Decentralization progresses slowly and is hindered by arguments of deregulation coming from central government. This problem will not be solved as long as it remains unclear which conditions will facilitate the optimal relation between decentralization and deregulation.

Another problem is the strong tendency towards bureaucratization and slow decision-making, which hinder or even obstruct the desired effects of cost control and the better manageability of the total health care system. It is necessary and possible to stop this tendency, but powerful participants will perceive such striving to be against their own interests. Total costs of health care are still rising, although at a slower rate than before 1974. It is not clear, however, whether this reduced rate of growth is caused by the new health policy or by the general retrenchment policy which developed in response to the economic recession.

Real cost control cannot be achieved as long as the nature of the financial system itself remains unchanged and as long as a gap remains between the planning and financing. Government only indirectly influences prices by the establishment of prior limits on tariffs. But the financial system itself, which contains many incentives to spend, has not changed. Doctors can compensate for lower tariffs by consulting more often, and indeed an increase in consultations has occurred during the last few years. The doctor's pencil is still the most expensive instrument in the whole health care system.

Moreover, the relations between planning, costs and financing are unclear. Whereas the planning decisions, taken under the Hospital Facilities Act, do determine hospital capacities, they fail to state the medical production to be obtained and the costs involved. Other problems arise because of the fact that the planning system must be decentralized, while the financing system is centralized. The trend to unbalanced growth is still perceivable, but seems to be less strong than before.

Furthermore, although the expansion of the in-patient sector has clearly slowed, only a limited reduction of in-patient capacity (number of beds) has occurred. The Netherlands remain characterized by a very strong in-patient and a very weak out-patient sector, despite all pronouncements of central government concerning the need to strengthen the out-patient sector. These shortcomings, namely, growing government interference, slow decision-making, the misfit between planning and financing and a trend towards unbalanced growth, have been discussed extensively, leading to the conclusion that cost and supply control were not being successfully implemented. As a reaction to that, the government appointed an advisory committee on the structure and financing of health care, presided over by a well-known captain of industry. The committee's report (Commissie Structuur en Financiering Gezondheidszorg 1987) was based on two ideas. Firstly, the insurance system had to be simplified. The second idea was less government and more market. As a consequence the Health Services Act has had to be withdrawn. In its latest reaction to the committee's report (Verandering verzekerd 1988) the government agreed on its essentials. Nevertheless it is still uncertain how the new system is going to be implemented. The original goals of the Memorandum of 1974 have not been reached, as is shown above. But this does not mean that there has been no effect at all. For instance, the legislation has brought about a number of changes in the quango structure. In 1982 the National Health Council succeeded the Central Health Council (instituted 1956) and the Central Organization for Health Tariffs replaced the Central Organization for Hospital Tariffs (instituted 1965).

Table 4.2 *Average percentages of seats for interest groups on Dutch health care quangos*

	Before 1982	After 1982
Health care institutions and medical professionals	39	39
Financing bodies	24	19
Employers	5	9
Employees	5	9
Consumers	0	4

Table 4.2 shows the average percentages of seats for each interest group before and after 1982. These comparative figures reveal a slight decline in the share allotted to financing bodies, and a small increase in the share allotted to organizations of employers, employees and consumers. This change is the result of a reduction in the number of seats occupied by the financing bodies in the Central Organization for Health Tariffs and the Council of Hospital Facilities. At the same time the financing bodies have strengthened their foothold in the National Health Council. Organizations of employers and employees, which were not represented in the Central Health Council and the Central Organization for Hospital Tariffs, do have seats in their successors. Opportunities for influence are now a little more evenly divided among various

interest groups. But there remains a heavy bias toward the organizations of health care institutions and medical professionals, with a corresponding disadvantage for the organizations of employers, employees and consumers. The financing bodies are somewhere in the middle.

The growth of the government's powers since 1974 certainly had an impact on the system, but did not cure all its ailments. In fact, some grew worse. One important reason for that is the fact that the use of these powers is restricted by the quangos, which all retain important tasks in the preparation and implementation of health care policy. Hence health policy-making in the Netherlands is controlled not only by the government but also by a number of interest groups which influence decision-making in this field. The concept of 'consociational corporatism' accurately labels this phenomenon. The dominance of the medical interest group can be explained as a consequence of the long existence (over 100 years) of a very strong medical professional organization, which maintains important lines of formal and informal influence over health policy-making. It is not at all certain that the newly proposed market-minded and deregulatory policy will bring about the changes needed. In 1988 everything seems to be in flux. It may well be that in ten years' time we will perceive that the 1987 report, like the Memorandum of 1974, marked the dawn of a new era. That may be, or it may not. As we remarked before, making plans is one thing, getting them implemented is quite another.

Note

Since no authorized English translation of the names of many health-related laws and organizations exists, the following list clarifies Dutch usage:

Algemene Wet Bijzondere Ziektekosten (AWBZ): General Special Sickness Expenses Act
Centraal Orgaan Tarieven Gezondheidszorg (COTG): Central Organization for Health Tariffs
Centraal Orgaan Ziekenhuistarieven (COZ): Central Organization for Hospital Tariffs
Centrale Raad voor de Volksgezondheid: Central Health Council
College voor Ziekenhuisvoorzieningen: Council of Hospital Facilities
Nationale Raad voor de Volksgezondheid: National Health Council
Structuurnota Gezondheidszorg: Memorandum on the Structure of the Health Services
Wet Tarieven Gezondheidszorg (WTG): Health Tariffs Act

Wet Voorzieningen Gezondheidszorg (WVG): Health Services Act
Wet Ziekenhuistarieven (WZT): Hospital Tariffs Act
Wet Ziekenhuisvoorzieningen (WZV): Hospital Facilities Act
Ziekenfondsraad: Sickness Fund Council
Ziekenfondswet (ZFW): Sickness Fund Insurance Act

5

The Politics of Health Reform: Origins and Performance of the Italian Health Service in Comparative Perspective

Maurizio Ferrera

According to the historical tradition of Western European continental countries, until the second half of the 1970s Italy's health system resembled the social insurance model, that is one based on a multiplicity of occupational schemes administered by relatively autonomous quasi-governmental funds (*casse mutue*). As a result of numerous coverage extensions three main types of insurance scheme had emerged: a general scheme insuring all employees of the private sector and their dependants (since 1943); a number of special schemes for public employees, for the self-employed and for particular occupational categories (founded partly between the wars and partly during the 1950s and 1960s); and a special scheme insuring against tuberculosis (since 1921). These schemes provided cash benefits and direct health care by means of contracts with doctors, hospitals, pharmacies, and so on. Regulations varied in terms of the range of benefits offered and their quality (Ferrera 1984, 1986).

In 1978 a sweeping reform led to the establishment of the Servizio Sanitario Nazionale (SSN), a single unitary scheme covering all citizens and replacing all previous schemes (except that for tuberculosis). The SSN has taken over the provision of all health care benefits which are offered free of charge (or with a small fee) to all citizens. All special regulations have been abolished. The 1978 reform also profoundly changed both the financing and the overall administration of the public health sector by suppressing all the *casse mutue* and conferring extensive organizational power on the regions and local governments.

How did the health reform come about? What political dynamics could lead to an institutional innovation of such vast scope? There is little need to underline the importance of these questions. With rare exceptions (typically the British reforms of the late 1940s and, to a lesser extent, the restructuring of the Scandinavian welfare states during the 1950s and 1960s) welfare reform has proceeded slowly through incremental adjustments, highly constrained by the pressure of countervailing forces. This has been especially true for the health field, which is characterized by a dense constellation of actors with diverging interests. Institutional incrementalism has in fact been the prevailing mode of change in all sectors of the Italian welfare state. The 1978 reform thus constitutes an interesting departure from national as well as international styles of social policy development.

This chapter will examine comparatively the political syndrome which allowed this departure. The first section will identify the constellation of actors most likely to influence the politics of health reform in developed welfare states and will then sketch a brief profile of the interactions among these actors in a number of countries. The second section reconstructs the politics of Italian health policy since World War II by describing the emergence and consolidation of the reformist coalition and its struggle against the counter-reformist front, until the final success of 1978. The third section sketches an overall profile of the Italian experience by raising some general questions of a comparative nature and discussing some of the major achievements as well as shortcomings of the SSN at work.

The Comparative Background

In describing the evolution of the Swedish health system, Heidenheimer (1980: 121) identified (with Dantean expression) three 'discs, intersecting on a common hinge, each of which supports a distinct set of structures: the political administrative disc; the professional education and status disc; the health care delivery disc'. Health systems are thus complex arenas composed of many different actors located on these different discs. In recent years a growing body of literature has explored the intricate interactions which take place in this arena. The aim has been to identify those tensions and alliances which accompany major reforms, particularly when broad institutional changes substantially modify the rules of the game, extending the scope of public regulation over market actors and forces (Alford 1975; Altenstetter 1974; Elling 1980; Glaser 1978; Heidenheimer 1973, 1980; Stone 1980). On the basis of this literature, health reforms can be analysed in terms of the power relationships among political parties (*per se* and as occupants of representative institutions), the medical profession, the bureaucracy (especially that segment responsible for health affairs), and local jurisdictions (especially in those countries where the constitutional framework or administrative tradition gives them special authority in the health field).

Left-wing parties everywhere tend to favour *étatiste* developments by promoting the extension of compulsory insurance, strengthening public regulation and curbing medical autonomy. Centre and conservative parties tend on the contrary to be more cautious and sensitive to private interests. Although they have also contributed to the expansion of the public side of the system when holding office, they have been more respectful of liberal principles of professional autonomy and market choice. Jealous of its own *esprit de corps* and of its socio-economic status, the medical profession generally defends the market orientation of the system (or at least public financing of private practice) from which it draws conspicuous benefits. Bureaucrats display more ambiguous interests. On the one hand, by nature they tend to oppose any alteration of the hierarchical status quo and of administrative routines; on the other hand, they occasionally manifest an interest in expanding their own resources and powers through an extension of public regulations and interventions. Centre–periphery relations may finally disturb the game of alliances among the previous actors and normally influence institutional outcomes in terms of centralization or decentralization.

This checklist of actors may certainly seem oversimplified if one is interested in explaining specific decisions or particular aspects of a given reform. However, an analysis of the power network among the actors mentioned can reveal a great deal if the aim is simply to understand the features of the macro-institutional framework (the public/private mix and, subsidiarily, the centralized/decentralized structure) of the health system in a given country or at a given time.

The balance of powers among these actors has historically tended to display only slow, marginal alterations. Institutional change normally follows an incremental path of gradual adjustments which largely reflect oscillations in the distribution of power. The experience of several European countries shows, however, that the balance may in some instances shift markedly in favour of a single actor. If, for example, leftist parties hold office and promote the socialization of medicine, pervasive institutional changes can occur, such as the establishment of a national health service or the transformation of doctors into salaried employees.

United Kingdom

Post-war Britain constitutes a paradigmatic example. The components of the political syndrome which replaced the sickness insurance system introduced by Lloyd George in 1911 with the National Health Service (NHS) can be summarized as follows:

1 The gradual weakening of the British Medical Association, largely hostile to the reform but torn by internal strains and profoundly dissatisfied with the existing system (particularly because of the contrasts with the friendly and other approved societies)
2 A strong Labour Party at both electoral and parliamentary levels, highly committed to welfare ideals (in a climate of intense, war-induced national solidarity) and backed by strong unions
3 A 'neutral' bureaucracy, relatively depoliticized but partly sensitive to union pressures
4 Weak local jurisdictions whose involvement in health affairs was strongly opposed by the medical profession.

The emergence of favourable conditions for the establishment of the NHS can be attributed to the marked weakness of one of the relevant actors as much as to the particular strength of any other. The fourth condition largely explains the centralized orientation of the original NHS until its 1974 reorganization (Klein 1983a; Levitt 1977; Watkin 1979; Willcocks 1967).

Sweden
The 'silent socialization' of the health system in Sweden originated amid a somewhat different political constellation of forces (Heidenheimer and Elvander 1980). After World War II the association of Swedish doctors (SMA) was stronger and more cohesive than its British counterpart. Thus it was able to resist the first serious attack on professional self-government and private practice represented by the Hojer reform plan. The proposals of a commission chaired by the director of the Board of Health, Axel Hojer, recommended a broad reorganization of the Swedish health system through wide delegation of responsibilities to the counties, an increase in the number of district physicians, and the establishment of a fixed schedule for doctor's fees (Serner 1980).

During the 1950s and especially the 1960s the SMA underwent a process of internal division owing to the increasing aggressiveness of younger doctors. The reformist wave of the 1960s culminated in the 'seven crowns' reform of 1970 which almost completely socialized Swedish medicine. That reform was made possible by an 'iron alliance' among the other three actors: the Social Democratic Minister of Social Affairs, the hospital authorities of the major municipalities, and the Federation of County Councils. The debts that the Social Democratic government owed to its allies in the struggle to tame the medical profession were paid through a considerable expansion of resources for hospital care and extensive decentralization of the health jurisdiction to the counties.

United States

If Britain and Sweden show how the balance of powers may in some cases shift in a direction favourable to socializing reforms, the United States constitutes a typical counter-example. Repeated attempts to introduce compulsory health insurance all failed, and the only significant innovations have been the (limited) programmes of Medicaid (for the poor) and Medicare (for the aged) in 1965. American doctors transformed their professional association (the American Medical Association or AMA) into an organizationally cohesive and politically aggressive centre of power. Its strong ally was the network of private insurance companies. By contrast, however, American political parties have always been much weaker and more permeable on the organizational level and much less committed to welfare objectives on the ideological level than European reformist parties. Finally the federal structure, extreme fragmentation and overlap of local jursidictions have considerably reduced the structural relevance of the other two actors. Thus the potential emergence of anything that could even vaguely resemble a coalition for health reform was improbable (Ehrenreich and Ehrenreich 1970; Glaser 1978; Marmor 1973; Starr 1982).

Continental Europe

In the countries of continental Europe, the equilibrium among the main actors of the health arena has tended to be more stable and balanced, thus leaving little room for the introduction of grand reforms or, in a negative direction, for the boycotting of a gradual but still increasing extension of the public hand. It is true, however, that some countries have displayed visible strains at certain times which have caused a substantial alteration of the distribution of power. For instance the Debré reform of 1958 and the social security reform of 1967 in France conspicuously curbed the traditional strength of the medical profession (Rodwin 1982). But such episodes have been relatively isolated and of limited relevance for comparison with North European reforms. In other continental countries a general consensus has tended to reinforce the status quo or at most to support only marginal adjustment. In Germany the institutional framework created at the end of Allied occupation has been approved by all actors and the issue of socializing reforms has never acquired a political saliency, not even within the SPD

(Altenstetter 1974; Leichter 1979). The great continental exception, then, is represented by Italy.

Although very brief and rough, this comparative survey suggests where one must look in order to find an explanation for the Italian phenomenon.

The Politics of Italian Health Policy

Historical and sociological studies on the evolution of the Italian health system are few in number. The reconstruction presented here is mainly based on works by Berlinguer (1973, 1979), Delogu (1967), Francesconi (1978), Freddi (1984b) and Piperno (1983, 1984, 1986). The post-war history of Italian health policy can be subdivided into three distinct phases.

The first phase started in 1948, with the new centrist coalition rejecting a reform plan drawn up by a parliamentary commission. The plan had recommended a thorough restructuring of the social security system which included the extension of health insurance to all workers, pensioners and dependants. During the 1950s the health sector developed in a fragmented and uncoordinated way through the proliferation of separate professional funds under strict control of the Christian Democratic Party (DC). By the end of the 1950s the *casse mutue* had become a major pillar of the Italian welfare state. The establishment of the Ministry of Health in 1958 did not substantially curb their powers. As was said at the time, the real minister was not the person sitting in the cabinet but rather the president of INAM, the largest *cassa* insuring all private employees.

The doctors were the strongest allies of the DC and, although in principle opposed, actively participated in the system of public health insurance. The government guaranteed their private professional status and lured them into acceptance by means of generous monetary and normative rewards. Relying on the Catholic background and orientation of most doctors, the DC allowed them to share in the health spoils such as posts on the hospital boards and other health agencies. Doctors even acted as patrons in the vote relationship, especially in the south and the countryside.

While the left opposition was active, its influence was minimal. At its 1956 Congress, the Communist Party (PCI) demanded a thorough reform of the health system which largely repeated the proposals of the 1948 parliamentary commission. At the same time the Socialist Party (PSI) was gradually elaborating the idea of a national pension and health insurance. In 1957, the leftist union CGIL submitted draft legislation for the establishment of a national health service, the first to be presented to parliament. In 1959 CNEL (a composite organ which represented the views of the top levels of ministerial bureaucracy and part of the academic intelligentsia) timidly proposed a universal extension of hospital insurance, but immediately qualified this by warning of the financial burdens involved. The idea of a health reform was slowly but tangibly gaining ground.

The centre-left coalition of 1962 opened the second phase of the history of Italian public health. The theme of health reform occupied a top position in the first planning documents prepared by the Republican (PRI) and Socialist (PSI) Parties. In 1963 CNEL publicized its plan for a reform of the social security system, which contained a fuller formulation of its 1959 proposal coupled with a comprehensive rationalization of the health funds. From their now stronger position, the unions renewed their pressures on the government; and in 1965 the PCI submitted its own reform proposal for a national health service. In the same year, parliament approved the first five-year plan prepared by the socialist Minister for the Budget, Giolitti, and approved by the entire centre-left cabinet. The plan explicitly committed itself to a national health service and the socialist Minister for Health, Mariotti, subsequently drafted a more concrete proposal. Conditions seemed to favour the establishment of a national health service; but this was not entirely the case.

The plan (especially its health section) was the object of heated debate. The Republicans, the Bank of Italy and CNEL all expressed serious misgivings about the financial aspects of such a development. But it was the DC in particular that withheld support, under pressure from the health funds' bureaucracy, the doctors and, less overtly, the entrepreneurs. Though not openly opposing the idea of a national health service, the DC tried to apply a very restrictive interpretation to this notion. That is, rather than being a broadly decentralized national insurance system to replace the health funds, it would complement them through a national agency charged with prevention, coordination and sanitation controls. At most, the DC was prepared to accept a rationalization of public health insurance by fusing the numerous existing funds into three larger health funds (*supermutue*) to cover private and public employees and the self-employed respectively.

The attempt by the DC to guarantee the survival of the *mutue* was obvious. During the first half of the 1960s, owing to the changing political and institutional climate, the latter had gradually been weakened. As a member of the coalition, the PSI was particularly influential in the Ministry of Health; autonomous regions were active in the health field and the centre-left coalition was committed to establishing ordinary regions, to which the constitution entrusted jurisdiction over health policy. Acting through the DC, the health funds were thus strenuously fighting to regain and preserve their institutional and political strength; they fiercely opposed any reform plan which would restrict their competence, let alone abolish them.

The doctors viewed the establishment of a national health service as a serious threat to their professional autonomy and economic privileges. Although none of the reform plans (and certainly not the governmental one) envisaged the transformation of doctors into salaried employees, the medical associations denounced the 'manoeuvre to nationalize the profession' and submitted a memorandum to CNEL in which they thoroughly criticized the Mariotti plan. The opposition to the establishment of a national health service was then still quite strong and also included the right-wing parties and the entrepreneurial associations (especially the pharmaceutical industry).

If the reformist front was still too weak to impose a national health service, it was strong enough to impose a hospital reform in 1968. This thoroughly revised the institutional setting and operating procedures of hospital care. The interest constellation was in this sector quite different from that of ambulatory care. The state of the Italian hospital system had continually deteriorated during the 1960s owing to the increasing demand for care. Still formally considered to be charitable institutions enjoying relative autonomy, hospitals were run according to strict principles of medical hierarchy. Even 'neutral' organizations such as CNEL had proposed a thorough revision of their status.

Change was also in the interest of counter-reformers. The financial situation of the health funds had deteriorated owing to increasing hospital costs over which they had little control. Budget deficits had already reached the worrying level of 250 billion lire by 1965 and had doubled to 500 billion by 1967. Within the medical profession itself, the number of younger doctors was rapidly growing owing to the opening of medical schools. Younger doctors had a more modern and socially oriented outlook; but above all, they resented the hierarchical status quo which did not allow them sufficient career prospects or even security of job tenure. Unionization levels increased markedly within their ranks, and pressure for a democratization of hospital structures rapidly mounted. These trends produced strains within the medical component of the hospital sector (Freddi 1984b). The status quo coalition thus had little cohesiveness because one of the partners (the *mutue*) was financially weak, while another partner (the medical profession) was riven by internal conflicts.

Given this situation, a concrete bargain could be struck on a reform in which all actors expected some gain. The left parties and the unions saw it as a first step after a series of long and frustrating debates and as an important improvement *faute de mieux*; they also hoped to gain new support from social strata which had traditionally been rather distant (such as doctors and paramedical staff). The health funds needed financial relief and were prepared to change the situation. Doctors (and more generally health workers' unions) hoped to gain power and jobs. Provided that a few 'vital' conditions were met (such as the protection of private and Catholic clinics), the DC was not opposed to a reform from which it hoped to draw fresh spoils to spend on the vote market. The electoral deadline completed the process, and in February 1968 the law was passed to everybody's satisfaction. The 'only small inconvenience of it', as an observer has subsequently put it, was that 'hospital costs tripled in only five years' (Salvati 1981: 11). The hospital reform marks the end of the second phase.

The third phase was characterized by the entry of new and powerful actors: ordinary regions, whose councils were first elected by popular vote in 1970. The birth of the regions greatly strengthened the constituency for the national health service. Immediately after their establishment, the regions initiated a fight against the central administration in order to force it to accomplish the transfer of functions (primarily health policy) foreseen by the constitution. This transfer offered a unique institutional and political opportunity for a thorough reorganization of the health system, the abolition of the health funds and the establishment of a national health service. Not surprisingly, however, resistance to this idea was slow to wither away. The regional elections had revealed the much feared strength of the left in local government which had resulted in the appearance of some 'red regions'. In this context, a health reform was not merely a matter of funds, doctors and costs; it was also a political question of prime importance, involving the 'gift' (or the 'conquest') of substantial resources for the opposition.

Thus central government (but again especially the DC) attempted a last defence of the health funds which, now largely as a result of the regulation introduced in 1968, were experiencing critical financial difficulties. The plan was to transfer hospital assistance to the regions, and thereby relieve the health funds of their most costly burden while simultaneously delaying the transfer of assistance and postponing *sine die* the liquidation of the *mutue*. The plan was supported by the smaller centre parties which, although not particularly in favour of the health funds, were concerned about the spending capacity of the regions.

Nevertheless, owing to the strength of the reformist front, the plan failed. The unions, regions, the left (especially the PCI) and the overall social and political temperature of the early 1970s together created such pressure for reform that in 1974 a law was passed which contained extraordinary provisions to repay the hospital deficit, transfer jurisdiction on hospital assistance to the regions, and (the most disputed point) fix a deadline of June 1977 for the definitive liquidation of the health funds. This law was the result of one of the most heated parliamentary struggles of the whole history of the Italian welfare state.

Not long thereafter the government submitted its own reform proposal for a national health service. The parliamentary proceedings lasted four years, not only because they were interrupted by the anticipated end of the legislature, but also because every actor was fighting to maximize gains. The PCI which, without holding ministerial posts, became a member of the majority coalition in 1976, visualized the national health service as a 'socialist reform in a capitalist setting' and pressed for decentralization and democratic (that is union/party) participation. The DC fought to limit the extent of the 'nationalization of health' and to preserve the status of private clinics and institutions, as well as the professional character of medical services and the level of practitioners' fees.

CNEL and the smaller centre parties were among the few who tried (and failed) to equip the reform with some adequate tools to stimulate and control economic and administrative efficiency. In December 1978, 21 years after the first reform proposals, with the support of all parties partaking in the national solidarity coalition (extended to the PCI), the Italian parliament approved law 833, establishing the first national health service of continental Europe.

Conclusions: the SSN at Work

Although very sketchy, this reconstruction of the main phases of Italian health policy identifies the most salient factors in the political syndrome which produced the 1978 reform. These four factors can be summarized as follows.

The first was the marked strengthening of the major party of the Italian left, coupled with the profound social and cultural upheavals of the 1970s. The growth of the PCI and its quasi-inclusion in the governing coalition greatly enhanced the potential for reform. Not only was this party ideologically committed to the SSN, but also it had acquired a prime political interest in its implementation; the health reform in fact transferred substantial assets but very few liabilities to regional governments, and many of these were dominated by the PCI.

The second was the gradual weakening and fragmentation of the medical profession. After the mid-1950s, ambulatory physicians became progressively bureaucratized as they subordinated themselves to the *mutue* system in exchange for economic and normative incentives, despite lip service to the sacred principles of free medicine. The medical profession lost its capacity for self-government and for professional assertiveness in matters regarding the organization of service delivery and the direction of medical training. The crumbling of the traditional hierarchical structure within the hospital sector and the mobilization of younger doctors destabilized the other relevant component of the profession. Bureaucratized and fragmented, Italian doctors could only serve as 'stone guests' in the public debate which accompanied the reformist wave of the 1970s. In practice they delegated to the Catholic Party the entire task of defining and defending their interests.

The third was the organizational and especially the financial disarray of the health bureaucracy, which gradually eroded the credibility and viability of the *mutue*.

The final factor was the establishment of ordinary regions. This was perhaps the most decisive event because it set an institutional obligation for a broad structural reorganization, raised the stakes of all actors (providing new stimuli especially to political parties), and originated a horizontal alliance (periphery versus centre) which cut across and thus further weakened the vertical counter-reformist alliance.

At this stage it may be premature to venture into a close comparison between the Italian experience and those of other countries. A thoroughgoing comparative explanation of the emergence of the SSN would require not only a fuller reconstruction of national events, but also more detailed information about developments in those European countries sharing with Italy a common welfare tradition. The relevant question would be why similar backgrounds have produced different institutional outcomes. In particular, a comparison between Italy and Germany might produce interesting results, since during the 1950s the two countries built fairly similar health systems; both were grounded on administrative backgrounds which had been heavily moulded by an authoritarian regime. How could the German system consolidate and prosper? How did it combine (rather successfully, it would seem) professional autonomy and financial and administrative viability with relatively high standards of performance in a context of growing public control of health care? What specific factors account for the gradual erosion of the Italian structure, and especially of its medical and bureaucratic pillars?

Another potentially informative comparison would contrast the North European and Italian paths to a national health service. The relevant comparative question would be why different historical and administrative backgrounds have produced similar institutional outcomes. With respect to Britain and Sweden, there are *prima facie* both remarkable elements of affinity (such as the weakness of the medical profession and the role of local jurisdictions) and remarkable elements of diversity (the extreme disarray of the health bureaucracy and their 'iron alliance' with the counter-reformist party; the presence of both a Catholic and a Communist Party). The task of future research will be to assess more carefully the weight and relevance of all these elements, with respect to both the preconditions and the institutional outcomes of the reform.

A close comparison with Britain and Sweden would not only cast new light on the specific syndrome which led to the *emergence* of the Italian SSN, but would also (and perhaps especially) allow an assessment of its *performance*. What are the most salient features of the new SSN, and how does it actually function with respect to its North European counterparts?

A decade from its establishment, the balance sheet of the new Italian service seems highly negative (Cavazzuti and Giannini 1982; Ferrera and Zincone 1986; Freddi 1984a; Piperno 1986). The only undisputed achievements are the universalization of entitlements to health care (thus filling the serious coverage gaps of the previous social insurance system) and the standardization of benefits and services (thus abolishing the high and absurd disparity of treatment across socio-economic categories).

The list of shortcomings is unfortunately much longer. Among the major indictments are the persistent resort to private provision of publicly financed services; the failure to reorient the health system from high-cost, hospital-centred care to more cost-effective community care emphasizing sanitation and prevention services; the irrational system of extremely centralized financing and extremely decentralized expenditure, coupled with inefficient devices of demand regulation; and the massive penetration of parties into the current management of the services.

Given the heterogeneity of the coalition which supported the reform, the original constitution of the SSN paid lip service to both the socialization of health and the concepts of professional autonomy and free choice. With these premises, nobody would have expected an evolution towards quasi-public medicine of the Swedish sort and very few saw this objective as desirable. It was hoped, however, that the reform would produce a transparent and rational mix between public and private, with a clearer definition and delimitation of these respective spheres. Many regarded the British system as an adequate approximation to the ideal mix. It was hoped that most non-ambulatory care could be provided by well-equipped, well-staffed and efficient public facilities while the private sector would retain a supplemental function in cases of extra-ordinary needs or in response to individual (and largely self-financed) preferences. Contrary to these hopes, the situation which has emerged is an ambiguous system of almost complete socializ-ation of costs plus extensive resort to private provision, especially in the grey but crucial area which lies between ambulatory and hospital care. Most services at this level are contracted out to private clinics and small diagnostic centres; public authorities have little control over the fees and over the referral system in these cases, and over-consumption and even fraud seem widespread. As in other sectors of the Italian welfare state, the ambiguous mixture of state and market has produced perverse incentives for an inefficient use (and often waste) of resources.

An overall reorientation of the health system which would give high priority to prevention services, community care, and specific target groups such as children, mothers, the aged, and the handicapped was one of the first and major aims of the 1978 reform. The reformers were particularly proud of this aim, which was seen as a sort of Archimedean point for restructuring the public health sector according to more advanced, North European criteria. Little has, however, been actually implemented in this direction. Apart from some pilot initiatives exclusively concentrated in developed areas of the north and centre of the country, the improvement of community care and the strengthening of prevention have remained mere wishes. The share of resources absorbed by institutional, hospital-centred care has actually been increasing since 1978 and had reached about 50 percent of the aggregate public health budget in 1985. Despite laudable efforts by a few enlightened bureaucrats, health planning and targeting have not succeeded in muddling through parliament and local administration to any effective extent. Territorial disparities on any relevant dimension of care have also been increasing, and the reformist aim of equal access to and equal opportunity for care has utterly failed.

The efficient functioning of the service is greatly impaired by the absence of rational financial incentives (Brenna 1984). Expenditure decisions are decentralized to regional governments, local health units and, ultimately, to individual providers. Central government has virtually no capacity of planning and control and limits itself to footing the aggregate health bill. A primitive system of supervision of the prescriptive behaviour of physicians and some rationing devices for consumers have recently been introduced; but the vicious circles of open-ended public financing seems still at work (Ferrera 1985). A number of proposals to confer greater financial responsibility to the periphery have been put forward, but without success.

The collusion of politics and administration is the last and perhaps most dramatic shortcoming of the SSN. The reform has entrusted all direct management responsibilities to elective committees expressed by local authority councils. Career administrators have been subordinated to these committees, which are mainly formed on the basis of party recruitment and political considerations. Thus part-time politicians and peripheral party cadres with little or no technical expertise and managerial skills have found themselves governing the new apparatus, formally freed of any hierarchical, administrative accountability and only vaguely and directly responsible to the electorate at large. It is hardly surprising that the result of this institutional setting has been an unwise, chaotic and at times even fraudulent administration. Consumer representation and democratic control (with or without the mediation of political parties) are valuable ingredients of any public health system and are actually found in Britain, Scandinavia and the United States (Checkoway 1981). In no country other than Italy have the distinct tasks of democratic control and of management been entirely subsumed into a single elective organ exposed to such heavy and thoroughgoing party manipulations.

The Italian reform record is thus largely unsatisfactory. Some of the shortcomings mentioned must certainly be imputed to the original design of the law, which in many respects was incoherent and confused. Some others have emerged during the implementation phase, distorting those general and abstract aims which were commonly regarded as wise and desirable when the law was passed. On different grounds, all partners of the reformist coalition of the past decade now try to keep aloof from the *real* SSN and its problems and to disclaim responsibility for its degenerations. In the intellectual debate, a movement in favour of a 'reform of the reform' seems gradually to be emerging, but it remains to be seen if its proposals of rationalization (more efficiency, more weight to technical skills, greater and more effective impulse behind the 'good' objectives of the SSN) will be capable of attracting a new, sufficiently strong political coalition.

6
Physicians and the State in France

David Wilsford

Physicians once were harassed practitioners of dubious medicine. Then at the close of the nineteenth century, with great organizing and improvements in science and technology, physicians became prestigious dispensers of health. Physicians' successes were so impressive that everyone claimed a right to them. Through governments and labour unions, people obtained more and more access to health care. However, such increased access required that more and more money be paid to physicians and their helpers for health care services. Governments, labour unions and employers began to question the relentless increase in expenditures. Physicians came under attack. This chapter examines the process and progress of that attack in France.

Physicians' Strategic Political and Market Position

Like its counterparts in many countries, the medical profession in France was able to consolidate an important political and market position. This historical power would later make a countervailing force essential to control health care expenditures.

For most of the nineteenth century, however, physicians in both Europe and the United States enjoyed neither high incomes nor high status. Their market position was poor, so their political influence was minimal. Medical technology was primitive and physicians were generally no more successful at treating illness and disease than witches, travelling medicine men, faith healers and the like (Rothstein 1972; Starr 1982; Bungener 1984). Further, patients did not seek out physicians if they could not pay them, so medical incomes were low. Although the *objective* demand for health care was higher than in the twentieth century (given conditions of sanitation, for example), there was little *subjective* demand for health care.

With industrialization and the advent of a large middle class, individuals began to be able to pay physicians for their services. The subjective demand for health care services also increased (Hatzfeld

1971). But even if able to pay, the sick will not patronize physicians if services are not better than the witches, medicine men and healers. An interaction effects model explains the rise of the orthodox medical profession and the consolidation of its control over health care. Both patients capable of paying (a large or growing middle class) and a service worth buying (the technological advances of medical science) were present before physicians' incomes and social prestige increased. From roughly 1890 to 1920 the orthodox medical profession in France transformed itself from a mere competitor with other health care providers into a hegemonic force controlling most aspects of the health care universe: hospitals, research, teaching and pharmaceuticals.

Physicians' incomes rose dramatically again after World War II because the state in both Western Europe and the United States began to pay physicians to treat poor and aged populations. The state in Western Europe and large private insurers in the United States also paid for more health care for the middle and working classes (Kervasdoué and Rodwin 1981). Third parties – the state and private insurers – expanded markets for physicians, increasing their incomes. Markets also expanded and incomes rose because a new wave of technological advances in diagnosis and treatment rendered previously untreatable illnesses treatable and previously incurable diseases curable.

In the nineteenth century the French medical profession expended great efforts to organize as a guild which could limit entry into the profession. As with any guild, upholding standards and protecting members were twin objectives. Of course, scientific and techno-logical advances were indispensable to guild organizing because they provided the objective basis for claims of expertise and the need to control quality. The guild effect limited supply, and demand increased in two stages; first with the rise of a middle class, and secondly with the rise of the welfare state and with general techno-logical advances. Physicians, of course, should have favoured the welfare state, for it increased subjective demand. Medical incomes in the United States, for example, rose most rapidly after the establishment of Medicare and Medicaid. Nonetheless, organized medicine in England, France and particularly the United States opposed efforts to expand and generalize the availability of health care through national health services or national insurance schemes.

Welfare State Crisis and Health Care Spending

The perception of a welfare state fiscal crisis was not new to the 1970s. Policy-makers in France confronted the economic pressures of funding extensive public health care programmes throughout the 1950s (Jamous 1969) and the 1960s (Collins 1969), even as they made the system more comprehensive. French social security generated growing deficits starting in 1949, which were due almost entirely to increasing health care expenditures. Corrective measures instituted after 1951 included increased fiscal controls, stabilizing administrative costs, and higher contributions from both employers and employees to the health care regime (Dumont 1981: 199–207). Economic pressures and ideological preferences led to a complex set of reforms, first in 1960 and then in 1967. These both expanded coverage and attempted to rationalize administration and organization of health care to control costs.

The chronic problem of rising health care expenditures was aggravated by the onset of general economic crisis after 1974. In France, the rate of annual real growth in GDP from 1951 to 1974 averaged over 6 percent with an average annual inflation rate of about 5 percent. From 1974 to 1980, the French rate of annual real growth in GDP fell to just under 1 percent with an almost 14 percent annual inflation rate.

Despite this crisis, the cost of health care and physicians' fees continued to rise rapidly. In France, annual national medical consumption increased from 2.8 percent of GDP in 1950 to 7.0 percent in 1977 (Barral 1978). Hospital costs rose most rapidly: from 1.1 percent of GDP in 1950 to 3.5 percent in 1977, or from 39 to 50 percent of total French health care expenditures. By 1984 France spent 8.0 percent of GDP on health care. From 1950 to 1974, French medical consumption increased nearly sixfold from 6.7 billion to 37.4 billion constant francs. In the same period, the French population increased 20 percent.

The pressures of two oil shocks in the 1970s and subsequent economic crisis exacerbated the financial disequilibria of public health care programmes. An ageing population and costly development of medical technology caused health care expenditures to increase at a far greater pace than GDP growth rates. Further, the expansion and evolution of hospital facilities during the 1960s and 1970s increased operating costs, in a secular trend over and above increases in personnel salaries. Once built, hospitals must be used. Overbuilding and subsequent surplus capacity aggravated the fiscal problem. Moreover, hospital budgets in France were calculated by the Ministry of Health according to occupancy per bed per day, thus eliminating any incentive for hospital directors and physicians to reduce patient admissions or length of stay.

Medical markets are peculiar markets and as such cry out for but also make difficult external regulation. Such regulation comes from either the state or other third parties such as private insurers and' employers. But because the medical market is not a 'normal' free market, there are important limits to possible reforms.

In theory, a free market is organized by free flows of supply and demand. Supply increases or decreases in response to demand; prices rise and fall according to the momentary equilibrium between supply and demand. Prices cannot in theory remain 'too high'. When too much demand chases too little supply, new producers enter the market. Their competition – nothing more than an increase in supply – lowers prices overall. When too many goods are offered for too little demand, producers lose money and withdraw from the market, thus decreasing supply. Prices rise. The global result of a free market is in theory an efficient equilibrium of supply, demand and prices which serves the interests of both producers and consumers.

But medical markets depart from the free market model in numerous ways. Their basic consumer–producer relationship encourages consumption. In medical markets the actual consumer does not pay; nor does the actual payer consume. The consumer end of the consumer–producer relationship is split, so the price–quality relationship is broken. The consumer has no incentive to be sensitive to price. The payer has at best imperfect means by which to verify quality. It is also very difficult to measure demand, supply and efficiency in medical markets. Thus medical markets tend to keep costs high, aggravating fiscal problems, for there is no *self*-regulating mechanism equivalent to competition for the 'free' market. Medical markets limit in important ways the possibilities for health care reform, chiefly by enabling physicians to disperse and defuse political pressures for economic change. Further, the decentralization of medicine and the ethical nature of health make it difficult both to locate culprits of waste and to sanction them effectively. External regulation of medical markets – by nature not self-regulating – must be imposed. In France the countervailing force to physicians and the external regulator of medical markets is the state.

The Character of the French State

Economic pressures on those who pay for health care came from general economic crisis, the progress of medical technology and the peculiarities of medical markets. These economic pressures generate political pressures on physicians. But political success against continued increase of health care expenditures varies according to the structures and traditions of the state. The French state, in so far as its authority is concentrated in bureaucrats and bureaucratic departments, has a distinct advantage in politics over organized medicine. In France, the Rousseauian view of the general will and the public interest pits the state against all entities, like interest groups (for example medical associations), which embody or epitomize 'particular wills', or private interests. The French state plays an important initiating and structuring role in interest politics, and groups are reduced to a reactive posture.

Certain tactical advantages enable the French state to induce and constrain the behaviour of medical associations (and other interest groups) and thus circumscribe their influence. These tactical advantages include (1) the government's proposal and decree powers, (2) a legislature of limited powers, (3) a strong executive, (4) the tradition of powerful ministerial *cabinets*, (5) an extensive bureaucratic corps of homogeneous elite training, and (6) a judiciary of limited powers (Wilsford 1988).

First, the 1958 constitution gives the executive in France the pre-eminent position in law-making. The executive can intervene in the parliamentary process and it has extensive powers of decree. The government is the master of the legislative process in France. It fixes all agenda items and the order of their consideration in both the Assembly and the Senate. The government may also circumvent the regular committee process by invoking parliamentary consideration of the original text submitted by the government. The government itself, on the other hand, may amend any text being considered at any time. Executive decrees also permit the government to modify laws in many areas and are juridically binding. Laws modified by decree are often decades old. Decrees in France combine imple-mentation regulations and independent law-making. The 1958 constitution permits vast domains of policy-making to be regulated by executive decree.

Secondly, the 1958 constitution changed the French parliament from a transformative legislature, which places its own imprint on legislation, into an arena legislature, where forces come together to debate large issues (Polsby 1975). In the Fourth Republic, interest groups pressured parliament, especially individual deputies, because party discipline was weak. Some parties were little more than electorally organized interest groups. Interest groups and political parties also collaborated for electoral purposes. Poorly organized interest groups concentrated pressure on bureaucrats who in turn pressured the administration for them. Since 1958, interest groups must concentrate almost exclusively on ministers and bureaucrats. There is less collaboration between interest groups and candidates or political parties for electoral purposes (Meynaud 1962; Wilson 1983).

Thirdly, the president in the Fifth Republic enjoys a power base independent of the legislature, for he is directly elected for a seven-year term. Deputies' terms may last no more than five years. (Senators serve nine-year terms, but are elected indirectly: in law-making, the Senate is less important than the National Assembly.) The president may also dissolve the Assembly. In the Fourth Republic, parliament directed the state politically, whereas the Fifth Republic places paramount political control in the executive. This control is centred in the president. Until 1986, despite the prime minister's strategic position and wide range of duties, the president has controlled the cabinet in both its makeup and its action. The strengthening of the executive and the weakening of parliament by the 1958 constitution make the actions and decision-making of the French state more coherent and efficient.

The 16 March 1986 legislative elections gave a parliamentary majority for the first time in the Fifth Republic to a coalition of parties opposing the incumbent president. The 1958 constitution permits parliament to deny confidence to the government – that is, the prime minister and cabinet chosen by the president. In this case, the president's alternative to resigning – to avoid prolonged crisis – is to appoint a prime minister and cabinet acceptable to the opposing parliamentary majority. In the event, François Mitterrand, a socialist, chose Jacques Chirac, leader of the conservative neo-Gaullist party, as prime minister and charged him with formation of the government. Cohabitation changes some institutional relationships in the Fifth Republic and damages the president's strategic position because the centre of executive power shifts from the president to the prime minister. But cohabitation does not constitute a return to the Fourth Republic's parliamentary regime. The executive remains strong and independent.

Fourthly, the tradition of powerful ministerial *cabinets* focuses the political direction of French administration. The French ministerial *cabinet* is a cohesive decision-making and policing unit serving the minister and separate from functional units in the ministry. The French minister has great freedom to compose his *cabinet* as he wishes and its members work for him on changing tasks. They also check on heads of functional departments, or *directions*, to ensure that directors act in the minister's interest.

The ministerial *cabinet*, a mix of political and technical brains chosen by the minister, is designed to focus the minister's directives effectively. It also serves as the centre for interministerial bargaining. By contrast with the American state, where unclear boundaries of authority and fragmented power centres accentuate the difficulties of political direction of bureaucratic policy-making and implementation, the *cabinet* gives the French minister an instrument of focused control over bureaucrats. Further, the Fifth Republic presidential cabinet, or Conseil des Ministres, like its British and unlike its American counterpart, constitutes a generally effective decision-making team under the direction of the president (or the prime minister) and adheres to a doctrine of cabinet responsibility.

Fifthly, the French bureaucratic corps – especially in its higher incarnations, the *grands corps* – is characterized by homogeneous elite training. Further, many of its highest members combine administrative and political perspectives. Up to 90 percent of the ministerial *cabinets* – which are distinctly political – may be members of the *grand corps*. This bureaucratic corps, with its common training in the *grandes écoles*, is important because administrators – bureaucratic, political and the combination in the *cabinets* – share a common view of the role of the state, its mission and its options, even if there are different interests and conflicts over them from one ministry to another, from one *direction* to another or between a *direction* and a *cabinet*. The values, beliefs and expectations characteristic of a state tradition of authority affect bureaucrats' perceptions of their interests and of the state's interests. Indeed, such a tradition gives the state an interest that is definable and defendable. The idea of the state shared by bureaucrats who staff its positions shapes their judgement of where interests lie, which of these are compatible with the state's interest, and what types of conduct are appropriate to the administrative-political universe.

Finally, in conflicts with groups, the French state (like the British) enjoys an advantage which its American counterpart lost with *Marbury* v. *Madison*: a judiciary of limited powers without a tradition of judicial review. The Revolution strengthened the asymmetry between judiciary and executive/parliament even though citizen rights were specified in the Declaration of the Rights of Man: freedom of thought and expression, freedom to own property, freedom from arbitrary detention and the presumption of innocence until proven guilty. Article 2 proclaimed that the fundamental purpose of political organization was to preserve the individual's natural rights, including the right to resist oppression. But there were no provisions for judicial appeal when these rights were violated. In general, either the executive or the legislature as the sovereign incarnation of Rousseau's general will both determined the general interest and protected individual rights. But protecting individual rights was secondary. The sovereign power could proclaim that the general will, or public interest, overrides individual rights. In the Rousseauian view, rights – inalienable in the American vocabulary – are fosterers of disunity.

The 1958 constitution continues the French tradition of limited judicial review. A constitutional council can pass on the constitutionality of parliamentary laws, but the executive is not subject to review by it. Originally only the president, the prime minister and the presidents of the Senate and the National Assembly could refer questions to the Council. Later a provision was added permitting 60 deputies or 60 senators to submit cases. The organization and philosophy of the French judiciary illustrate the institutional relationships between the strong state and its citizens, whether as individuals or as interest groups. Limited judicial access and limited judicial powers give the state greater autonomy in its relations with civil society.

Medical Associations as Interest Groups

Medical associations exemplify certain strengths and weaknesses in the face of political and economic pressures. They are foremost *professional associations* with a common basis for organization and maintenance of the group. This advantage is based on common education and practice of a common profession with common values. Professionals also come into frequent and regular contact with their colleagues which reinforces their perception of a common interest. This contact occurs in law firms and with law practice, in medical practices and hospitals, in university departments and in professional meetings. Professional associations are also directly concerned with economic interests. The common basis of professions and practising a profession for economic reasons (physicians, lawyers and professors are all concerned with income and working conditions) make the economic incentive important to their daily existence. Finally, professional associations control the exercise of social and economic functions (for example, law, medicine, teaching) which make their success critical to citizens and to policy-makers.

Some interest groups are more strategically positioned in society and in the economy. For example, at the end of the nineteenth century organized medicine in France used science and technology to improve its strategic position. The subject of medicine – health – also provided a better strategic position to physicians, for health is generally considered more important to more people than, say, a university education. Thus physicians succeed more often in political action than professors, though both are professionals.

Two aspects of strategic position are environment and conjuncture. *Environment* contributes constraints or opportunities to specific interest groups. For example, the difference between an open and a closed policy-making arena affects the ease or difficulty with which a group may press its claims on the policy-making process. Groups enter open arenas more easily than closed arenas. But groups which dominate a closed arena enjoy greater opportunities to press their claims than groups outside the arena. Interest groups seek to keep arenas closed if they dominate, or penetrate closed arenas if they are excluded, or close open arenas in their favour (Wilsford 1984). In medicine, the scientific-technological imperative – with the rise of science and its applications to medicine – gave physicians an opportunity to close what had been an open policy-making arena in many countries, including France. Science and technology – environmental characteristics – permitted physicians to legitimize their claims to expertise. The economic advantages of securing professional sovereignty are obvious, but success in securing it depended on skill, creativity, intelligence and favourable environment – that is, making good use of an opportunity, which physicians did.

Conjuncture also contributes constraints or opportunities to interest groups. For example, in 1945 the post-war desire in Britain and France to ameliorate their pre-war records of social services was both a constraint and an opportunity of conjuncture. The medical profession's normally effective opposition to national health services or national health insurance was less effective because of this conjuncture. Similarly, groups opposed to liberal medicine enjoyed a greater opportunity to establish or expand national health care than before the war.

The difference between environment and conjuncture is analytically the difference between long- and short-term factors. Environmental constraints and opportunities for interest groups are more permanent. Conjunctural constraints and opportunities are more temporary. Long- versus short-term factors also mean that conditions favourable to or opposed to certain interest groups change more or less quickly. Environmental change comes about more slowly. Conjunctural change may be more rapid – but also more fleeting. Some conditions and some changes in strategic position may combine aspects of the two (Wilsford 1985).

Olson (1965) argues that no single member of the group is able to pay the full cost of organizing and maintaining the group, but also that no single member is incited to join or support a group if he will enjoy the benefits provided or obtained by the group without joining. Labour unions have thus always sought closed-shop agreements with management. Because of free riders, groups cannot take solidarity or incentives for collective action for granted. Yet all groups are not subject to the free rider problem to the same degree. Some solidarity and therefore more likely collective action exists in certain types of groups.

For professional associations, the profession provides a certain *a priori* solidarity. This solidarity is based on values, inculcated by common education (medical schools) and perpetuated by daily contact among members of the profession (hospitals and academic medical departments) and enforced by common sanctions (the ethics of medicine). From an economic perspective, professional sovereignty is also a mechanism for controlling supply and demand and therefore prices, and thus incomes and employment opportunities.

Yet professions are not relieved of the free rider problem. In France, according to government figures, of approximately 85,000 practising private physicians in 1984, 32,000 *at the most* were members of a medical association (well under 40 percent). Of these, the Confédération des Syndicats Médicaux Français (CSMF) was estimated to have 17,000 members, the Fédération des Médecins de France (FMF) about 9,000. Professional associations must work hard for members. Doing so means dealing in selective benefits: physicians need association meetings and the benefits of association journals. Both the CSMF and the FMF publish periodicals of news and professional information, and offer their members a series of postgraduate training programmes on such topics as social security, health care economics, communication and negotiating techniques, computer applications in medicine, and management of a private practice. The CSMF and the FMF together receive about 5 million francs per year subsidy from the government for these training programmes.

Because members are hard to organize and difficult to keep, medical associations have historically deployed resources in the pursuit of professional sovereignty. The licence monopoly and the prohibition of market competitive instruments such as advertising and mergers have been especially effective. Organized medicine is quick to decry any dilution of sovereignty once obtained. Free riders make protectionism important to medical organizing.

Cohesion and Fragmentation of the Medical Profession

The economic peculiarities of medicine and its markets give physicians a strategic advantage over the state and private insurers in health care politics. Physicians are masters of consumer decision-making in health care and market functions are extremely decentralized. Further, common education and ethics and the resulting professional bonds are important sources of cohesion for the medical profession. But sources of fragmentation also affect organized medicine. Competing sectoral and professional interests are characteristic of both French and American physicians. But French physicians are even more fragmented because of their tendency to organizational particularism.

Because physicians are members of a profession, they benefit collectively from numerous sources of cohesion. Professions are service occupations that apply a systematic body of knowledge to problems which are highly relevant to central values of the society. To become a member of a profession, a long socialization process is designed to build up technical competence and establish firm commitment to values and norms central to the tasks of the profession. Values and norms are further institutionalized by the structure and culture of the profession. Professional autonomy and cohesion are ensured by such practices as laws against quacks, professional referral patterns and norms which restrict certain forms of competition, insistence on exclusive professional competence in judging performance, and professional personnel in and professional advice to government agencies (Rueschemeyer 1964).

For medicine the profession's relation to society is characterized by an important consensus: everyone agrees on the broad definition of health and its importance. Both the patient's and the doctor's interests converge. Physicians can also claim the objectivity of science and – joined with high technical complexity – the sole authority to judge outcomes. This claim enhances professional cohesion.

But in medicine there is divergence of interests along other dimensions which are sources of fragmentation. Many different interests are common to health care politics: hospitals, physicians, nurses, private insurers, laboratories, pharmaceutical companies and medical equipment manufacturers. These interests often compete and their goals diverge.

Within the medical profession itself, intraprofessional divisions are often salient: generalists versus specialists, specialists versus each other, hospital physicians versus private practitioners, physicians versus surgeons. For physicians, the potential advantages of cohesion inherent in sharing a profession are often offset by the medical profession's dispersion, especially characterized by the solo practitioner. Association memberships are also often higher among specialists than among general practitioners. Specialists are more strongly tied together by their shared discipline and by their relatively small numbers. For example, the association of cardiologists counts 1,200 active members of 2,500 cardiologists in France, a membership ratio which far exceeds that of the general medical confederations combined. The numbers of generalists, on the other hand, and the extreme diversity of their geographical and professional situations tend to reduce their sense of cohesion and thus their participation in professional associations. These sociological factors work to keep physicians apart, and not only make it difficult to organize but also force them to attend to coalitions and strategic alliances.

The importance of intraprofessional divergence of interest is manifest in the French hospital system. Michèle Barzach, Minister of Health in the 1986 Chirac government, argues that 'today 35,000 hospital practitioners have completed 20 years of studies but have almost no career hopes. That's not normal. The people in charge have to change. We can no longer permit *chefs de service* to be named for life. We need five-year terms with an evaluation at the end, as is the case in the United States.' Despite misunderstanding the American context, Barzach points to a growing problem that divides the hospital corps. With the organization of French hospitals into fief-like services headed by a *chef de service* named by prefectoral decree for life, younger careers are blocked. Yet as medical demography gallops, the number of young physicians in the hospital system grows far more quickly than the number of hierarchical positions which open due to death or retirement. Thus even physicians within the same speciality fragment between mandarins on the one hand and their medical service staffs on the other.

Organizational Particularism of the Medical Profession in France

The French medical profession historically enjoyed a strong political and economic market position. Economic pressures on health care systems then led to political pressures on organized medicine. French physicians withstood these pressures less well than their counterparts elsewhere because they favour organizational particularism. American physicians, by contrast, favour organizational universalism. Because the one is formally fragmented while the other is formally unified, American physicians are more powerful than their French counterparts in the face of similar economic and political pressures. Through the AMA, the American profession has a centralized political structure. It faces a diffuse organization of responsibility for health care policy at all levels of Congress and the administration. By contrast, the French profession is diffusely organized and faces a centralized political structure in the state administration.

Particularism in France means that interest sectors are highly fragmented ideologically and non-ideologically. Such fragmentation provides the French state with many opportunities to structure interest-group politics. Groups within an interest sector are often distinguished not by function but by ideological politics. While less than 15 percent of the French industrial workforce is unionized, for example, at least three major labour confederations compete for members in each plant. Each confederation may be identified with a distinct ideological politics.

Physicians also fragment ideologically. In the small but influential subsector of medical professors, four associations – distinguished by ideological politics – compete to represent the subsector's interest. In addition to two mainly conservative confederations representing private practitioners (the CSMF and the FMF), there are also socialist and communist associations which claim to do the same. Indeed, there are no medical *associations* in France, only medical *unions (syndicats)*. The difference in terminology points to a more political defence of sectoral professional interests in France than in the United States with its ostensibly apolitical associations.

In France, because of particularism, dissident movements frequently leave the parent organization to form new, competing associations. During the 1960s, a schism within the CSMF led to the formation of the rival FMF. Both umbrella associations compete for members and for the government's attention, thus weakening the profession's influence. In France, there is no equivalent to the American Medical Association, a single umbrella organization uniting the entire profession for political (and other) purposes.

Medical Syndicalism in France

The oldest and largest medical association representing private practitioners in France is the CSMF. Founded in 1928, it had consolidated its pre-eminence by 1930. The CSMF employs roughly 40 full-time staff in its Paris headquarters, including full-time elected officials. It is made up of associations in 92 of 95 French departments (not counting overseas departments or territories). Departmental associations affiliate with the national CSMF. They are typically staffed by any elected president, an elected secretary-general, sometimes an elected treasurer, and a full-time secretary or two. Twenty-seven specialty associations are also affiliated in addition to the departmental associations. Twelve other groups, such as the Syndicat National des Médecins du Sport or the Syndicat National des Médecins de Groupe are loosely federated with the national office. The primary organizational principle of the CSMF is geographical or horizontal. Specialty or vertical organizing is secondary. The association claims more than 15,000 dues-paying members. Dues are approximately 1000 francs (roughly $150) per year to the national ôrganization and from 100 to 500 francs (from about $15 to $75) per year to the departmental associations. Specialty association dues tend to be slightly higher.

The roots of the CSMF lie in the beginnings of the medical syndicalist movement in France near the close of the nineteenth century. The first *syndicat médical* was formed in the Vendée in 1881. This region lies on the Atlantic coast between La Rochelle and Nantes. The union was illegal because French associational law at the time was based on the June 1791 Le Chapelier law forbidding any manner of association. The formal privileges of various professions were suspended. The practice of medicine was thus no longer protected, regulated or restricted. Rather, free enterprise ruled. The medical professions under the *ancien régime* were typical medieval guilds: hierarchical, closed monopolies. Physician guilds were thus a natural target of the revolutionary fervour against combinations contrary to the general interest. In 1884 workers' unions were legalized but liberal professions were not included.

The creation of the Vendée medical union exhibits characteristics common to all subsequent organization of physicians' interests in France. In the face of a strong and unyielding state, the syndical movement came from the grassroots and took the form of contestation. Between March and December 1881, eleven departmental unions were formed, but there were no formal ties between them. By 1884 there were approximately 150 departmental unions with a total of 3,500 physician members. In November 1884, 40 of these unions joined together to form the Union des Syndicats Médicaux de France (USMF). But a ruling by the circuit court of appeals (*cour de cassation*) on 27 June 1885, confirming two lower court decisions, declared the USMF illegal under the terms of the Chapelier law. The new law of 21 March 1884 permitting occupational unions did not apply to the liberal professions. While medical unions continued to exist and to form, not until the comprehensive law of 30 November 1892 were they declared legal by specifically extending provisions of the occupational unions' law to physicians. This 1892 law established both conditions of practice and penalties for malpractice. It also restricted activities: while physicians were permitted to unite in syndical organizations in defence of their interests, they were not permitted to exercise this right against the state, its departments or its communes.

After 1884, the USMF collectively represented the regional associations of physicians that had rapidly developed. Nevertheless, organizational particularism affected it in two ways. First, syndical organizers wanted another structure created within the profession but independent of the USMF to license and police the practice of medicine. Eventually the Vichy regime created the Ordre des Médecins in 1940 which, although reformed in 1945, still enforces the ethical code and administers licensing. Thus the French medical profession never combined the powerful disciplining and licensing prerogatives with union activities and representation, as did the AMA.

Secondly, the first but not last schism in French medical syndicalism occurred within the USMF between 1915 and 1928. In the course of a lengthy period of social policy-making that began with the return of Alsace and Lorraine to France and ended with the passage of the first comprehensive French health insurance system in 1930, two sides formed. On the one hand, USMF loyalists argued – in agreement with successive governments – that the adaptation of Alsace and Lorraine's comprehensive health care system to the rest of France should include such Bismarckian features as collective contracts between physicians and local sickness funds and third-party payment by the funds directly to physicians for their services. The dissidents based their opposition upon the four sacred principles of the 'Medical charter', tenaciously praised today by the French medical profession as at once holy and inalienable. These principles are (1) freedom of physician choice by the patient, (2) freedom of prescription by the physician, (3) fee-for-service payment, and (4) direct payment by the patient to the physician for services rendered. Together these principles constitute what the French call *la médecine libérale*. In 1926, dissidents established a rival to the USMF, called the Fédération des Syndicats Médicaux de France (FSMF). However, since the 1930 social insurance law included the four principles of the medical charter, the two organizations reunited under a name first used in 1928, the Confédération des Syndicats Médicaux Français.

During the occupation, Vichy dissolved unions and associations of every kind and replaced them with obligatory and unitary corporate bodies. The Ordre des Médecins regrouped all physicians into a single organization. The Order policed the practice of medicine and served as the policy conduit from the Vichy authorities to the medical profession. The officers of the Order were appointed by the government.

After the Nazi defeat, French unions and associations were again legalized in 1945. The Ordre des Médecins was reformed. More important, the social security system established in 1930 was completely replaced. The ordinance of 19 October 1945 instituted a new, expanded social security in three parts: retirement, family allowances and health care. The political impulse for this revised system came both from the widespread feeling that pre-war social services were indeed dismal and from the widespread suspicion that this state of affairs largely explained the 1939 defeat. An ideology of national solidarity underlay the post-war social security reforms.

French physicians generally favoured the national health insurance of the new social security system, but there were numerous details of dispute. The first major conflict with the post-war government was over setting fees. Originally, the Ministers of Labour, Health and National Economy were to fix fee schedules independently. Organized medicine – which had not been consulted in establishing the new social security and health care policies – objected. Parodi, the Minister of Labour and chief proponent of a new comprehensive social security system, chose to accommodate physicians' demands in order to forestall further opposition to his programme. He agreed to establish a tripartite commission, composed of equal parts of state authorities, sickness fund representatives and the medical profession, which would meet periodically to negotiate the fee schedules. The commissions would operate under the tutelage of the Ministries of Labour and Economy. Quasi-independent in theory, they were in fact closely dependent on the government, for the law permitted the government to set overall contribution and expenditure levels for the system. Throughout the 1950s the financial disequilibria of the social security system grew, despite corrective measures as early as 1950. Successive governments believed that one essential way of grappling with the fiscal problem was to contain physicians' fees.

In 1946, the government sought to establish a fee system *opposable* or binding on all physicians. In the French system, following the dictates of *la médecine libérale*, patients paid physicians directly and were later reimbursed specified amounts by the sickness funds – usually 75 to 80 percent of the scheduled fees. Hospitalization, however, was covered 100 percent and paid directly by the funds. Because the scheduled fees were not binding, percentages of reimbursement of fees actually paid by patients varied widely – sometimes as low as 30 percent of the fee charged. Without a binding schedule, physicians charged what they wished.

With the support of the sickness funds and both labour and management who administered them, successive governments sought a binding fee schedule. Two reasons proved equally compelling. First, the ideology of national solidarity, especially in the immediate post-war period, was widely shared. This sentiment cut across traditional ideological cleavages and traditional economic class divisions. Secondly, as physicians raised fees beyond those specified by the reimbursement schedules, sickness funds and successive governments came under pressure to raise the fees specified by the schedules.

Physicians fought a series of government attempts to establish binding fee schedules throughout the 1950s. The CSMF barely staved off a comprehensive initiative of the Minister of Social Affairs in 1956–7, and French medical syndicalism was forced into a reactive posture against the state. The CSMF leadership moved towards a policy of relative conciliation as most realistic, but two tendencies within the medical profession became evident. A large and growing dissident movement opposed cooperation with the government or the sickness funds in any new binding fee system. The tension between these two tendencies represented the difference between contestation from without versus contestation from within normal negotiating channels. Finally, the decree of 12 May 1960 imposed binding fee schedules negotiated at the departmental level on all physicians. Further, the decree permitted physicians to adhere individually to the negotiated agreements, thus eliminating one of organized medicine's most crucial roles as spokesman for and representative of individual members. Individual physicians who did not sign agreements to abide by these fee schedules lost their patients' rights to be reimbursed by the sickness funds. The French medical profession formally splintered as several dissident movements broke off from the CSMF to form their own organizations.

Numerous departmental affiliates and some specialty associations left the CSMF to form the Union Syndicale des Médecins de France (USMF). Others left to found the Association Médicale pour la Recherche et l'Union Syndicale (AMRUS). The Fédération Nationale des Géneralistes Français (FNMGF) was a third organization that claimed a national membership. In 1967, these three joined together better to oppose the CSMF and formed the Fédération des Médecins de France (FMF). From 1967 until 1985, a series of conflicts pitted the CSMF against the FMF over such issues as fee agreements, social benefits, and cooperation with state authorities. But in 1971 the state recognized the FMF as officially representative of the entire medical profession, in addition to the CSMF. It thus became the second privileged interlocutor of the government and the second official negotiator for physicians with the sickness funds.

The fission of French organized medicine into two competing national associations manifested itself in concrete ways over specific issues. In 1971, the CSMF signed the first negotiated national *convention* fixing physicians' fees; the FMF refused to do so. In 1976, the FMF was the only party to sign the second national *convention*, although both groups took part in negotiations. In 1980, the FMF alone negotiated and signed; the CSMF finally added its signature in 1981. On each occasion, the state decreed that because one organization representative of the entire medical profession had signed, the provisions of the *convention* would apply to all physicians. Only for the 1985 *convention* did both groups participate fully in the negotiations with the funds and approve the final product.

Consultation, Cooperation and Contestation

Relations between the state and organized medicine in France may be characterized by consultation, cooperation and contestation. The state draws medical associations officially into administrative decision-making through consultative bodies and advisory commissions. This kind of *consultation* legitimates administrative decisions and gives the medical associations the indispensable access to decision-making which they cannot otherwise be guaranteed. Because the administration has an upper hand over the arrangement of its relations with the medical associations, the associations must *cooperate*, especially when associations are in competition with each other because of organizational particularism. Nevertheless, the system is so weighted in favour of the administration that abuse is common. When associations decide they can no longer participate, they *contest* by exiting the administrative universe and engaging in some form of direct political action, such as boycotts, demonstrations or strikes. As one medical association president reported: 'You know, if the administration does not want to give us something we want, what else can we do?'

Consultation is frequent in France, much of it institutionalized in advisory commissions which meet regularly. Mignot and d'Orsay (1968: 92) estimated the number of commissions at over 15,000. Ehrmann (1983: 204) estimated that there were 500 councils, 1,200 committees and 3,000 commissions which bring together members of organized interest groups and the bureaucracy at the national level. Ehrmann notes that the Ministry of Finance alone consults more than 130 committees. In health care, dozens of commissions, councils and committees advise on policy-making: the Conseil Supérieur des Hôpitaux, the Conseil Supérieur d'Hygiène Public, the Conseil Supérieur de Médicament, the Conseil Supérieur de Pharmacovigilance, and so on.

The French state's tactical advantages and the particularist organization of interests enable the bureaucracy to 'consult' different interests as policy is formulated. This seemingly substantive input into decision-making is commonly called *concertation* in France. But such consultation is often superficial, for it enables the state to find support for its own view while ignoring or diffusing opposition.

Ministers and bureaucrats enjoy great discretion in deciding whom to consult and whom to listen to among the consulted. The state uses its tactical advantages to structure interest-group activity and policy outcomes by opening or closing policy-making arenas to different participants. One interest-group leader complained that too often even formal consultation is just that: formal but not substantive. This leader cited the example of discussing a proposed measure in a ministerial committee meeting and then seeing the final text of the measure printed the next day in the *Journal Officiel* (Wilson 1983: 900). According to one medical association leader: 'Of course, we and other medical associations were invited to the ministry. But in the end, and even during discussions, the outcome was clear. The government already had its mind made up and "listened" only to those groups which shared the government position.' Access does not necessarily equal influence. Consultation is often no more than a symbolic benefit.

Suleiman's respondents (1974: 333ff), for example, argued that consultation served an informative and persuasive function – *from* the administration *to* interest groups. 'My job is to explain and to inform . . . Contacts [with interest groups] are necessary. But I think I can say that we always manage to have our view prevail,' argued one director. Another reported: 'We always consult. It doesn't mean that we listen, but we consult. We don't always reveal our intentions. We reveal only as much as we think it is necessary to reveal.' Thus Suleiman argued that one important function of consultation is the opportunity it gives the administration to present interest groups with *faits accomplis*, that is decisions it has made before consultation.

Unlike the American practice of early consultation as proposals are formulated (Chubb 1983), consultation in France occurs late in the administrative decision-making process. In a typical policy process the preparation of texts – laws, decrees or reforms – begins in secrecy within a small administrative group. Gradually the initial group seeks the agreement and cooperation of other groups within the ministry and then from other ministries. Once a final text is agreed upon by the administration, interest groups are approached and informed of the proposed policy. A closed approach is essential, a director reported to Suleiman (1974: 335–6), 'because otherwise there will be opposition over every provision and the text will never get drawn up'. Another director commented: 'We ask for [interest groups'] advice only *after* we have a completely prepared text. And we do this just to make sure that we haven't made some colossal error' (1974: 336). In health care, one regional medical group leader lamented with evident frustration: 'We never know about anything until it's done.'

But medical associations are not fooled by these formalities of consultation. They realize that in normal politics the administration has an upper hand in policy-making and that their influence in the consultative process is often minimal. In reforms of medical education and hospital administration, conservative medical associations were regularly consulted by the Socialist administration. But in a curious paradox, both sides knew that conservative interest-group views would be certainly ignored by Socialist administrators. Why the minuet? Because the Socialists, like all administrators, were influenced by persistent hopes of forestalling opposition to reforms; likewise, conservative interest-group leaders were influenced by persistent hopes that their opinions might make a difference. In the end, consultation served no substantive purpose. The administration promulgated reforms; conservative medical associations organized demonstrations and boycotts. Abuse of consultation has reduced even its symbolic benefits.

To counter protest, administrative symbolism persists. The government may publicize symbolic concessions to protesting groups 'only to retract or deform them after the demonstrators have demobilized' (Wilson 1983: 906). When hospital interns were on strike, the government first satisfied their demand for restitution of prestige titles. Only when the strike continued and such symbolism proved insufficient to diffuse protest in a strategic policy area did the government satisfy interns' second demand for pay increases. The state's tactical advantages often enable it to retract or not implement concessions that are not symbolic.

In the face of an unresponsive administration, recourse to the judiciary can occasionally help. When some groups representing medical professors challenged the government's decree establishing elections to organize *conseils supérieurs* which control the nomination and promotion of university faculty, the Conseil d'État ruled illegal the decree's provisions for representation on the *conseils*. But the French judiciary is usually a less effective avenue of protest than in the United States. The legal avenue is more heavily circumscribed by the constitution in France, and a different ethic of the law and judicial review permeates French thinking. As one leader noted; 'We have no illusions about the effectiveness of legal action. We believe that the strength of the social forces is more influential and that it even influences the judges as they render their decisions' (Wilson 1983: 904).

Similarly, legislative support is generally useful only in the long term, for many decrees cannot be changed or can only be modified slightly. For example, a conservative medical association might lobby members of the Senate where the conservative opposition held its only majority from 1981 to 1986. But even if the association succeeds in getting a Senate vote opposing, say, Socialist reforms of medical education or hospital administration, the government under the Fifth Republic constitution decides which chamber's version prevails. Why go to this kind of effort? One medical leader answered: 'As a last resort. There was nothing else to do. And it is important to keep the opposition involved for when they return to power.'

Often an interest group's only effective recourse is direct action, such as boycotts, demonstrations or strikes. Hence there is a long history of direct action in the medical profession. From 1979 to 1985, a period including governments of both right and left, physicians demonstrated in May 1979, March 1982, June 1982, September 1982, April 1984 and February 1985. They struck in June 1980, spring 1983, November and December 1983 and January 1985. Hospital interns struck in March 1982, all of spring 1983, September 1984 and March 1985. Numerous boycotts punctuate relations between state and medical associations. For example, hospital physicians boycotted elections to the consultative commissions which were to implement departmentalization in 1985. In 1986, the CSMF decided to boycott health ministry advisory commissions until the government rescinded its plan to allow midwives to read echographs without the supervision of the attending obstetrician or gynaecologist.

But little evidence suggests that isolated or less than *massive* strikes or demonstrations influence the state. For example, hospital interns got symbolic concessions first, but had to wait on the crucial issue of pay. Problems in the departmentalization of hospitals plague the government. But in the end reform of medical education and hospital administration has proceeded about as planned. From the institution of the *convention* to the reorganization of the *internat*, the French state has been remarkably able to reform the health care system over the objections of the medical profession, although reforms sometimes cost more than originally planned. The French state places medical associations in a reactive posture.

Contestation, especially based on direct action, is of course a two-edged sword. One medical association president reported: 'I have a lot of trouble with my people in Strasbourg. They're always going on a wildcat strike. If I can't control my people, then the administration begins to think that I am not a worthy interlocutor. But it works both ways. As long as wildcat strikes don't happen too often, then sometimes they strengthen my hand with the administration.' Further, to call a boycott, demonstration or strike is fraught with uncertainty. It is difficult to be sure that members will participate fully. If they do not, a failed strike or demonstration reduces an association leader's influence with the administration.

In the array of contestation techniques, risk and cost vary. The least risky direct action is the boycott; if it fails, less is lost than if a demonstration or strike fails, which are riskier in that order. The organizational cost of these techniques also varies. The least costly is a boycott, the most costly is a strike. Nevertheless, each seeks to force the hand of the government and as such is riskier and more costly than 'negotiating' from within the administrative system.

Further, the utility of the strike to the medical profession – despite its widespread use by French physicians – is questionable. A strike must impose a loss on the employer. To do so, it must stop production. But a medical strike which stops production is not ethical, for physicians have defined their calling in such a way as to emphasize its humanitarian and indispensable character. Defining their calling that way gives physicians the logical basis for claims of exclusivity and quality control. Bound by moral codes, the medical profession can never strike in the same way as other occupations. Hence the prevalence of *grèves administratives*, or administrative strikes. In such a strike, physicians refuse to process paperwork, attend administrative meetings or otherwise facilitate the system's administrative functioning. *But they do not refuse to treat sick people.* Consequently, the effect of the strike is automatically minimized. Hence physicians frequently use demonstrations as a surrogate for the strike.

Relations between the French state and the medical profession are weighted in favour of the state. As we have seen, the 1960 *convention* was a system of fee agreements *imposed* on French physicians by the decree of 12 May 1960, against their bitter opposition. The new system divided the CSMF and led to the schism which produced the FMF. The 1970 *convention*, instituting fee negotiation by medical associations, was also established by decree. The 1976 and 1980 *conventions* were signed only by the FMF but were applied by the state to *all* physicians, despite the FMF's minority status. The state's tactical advantages enable it almost always to win its conflicts with physicians.

The state's central power over physicians is also manifest in its pivotal tutelage over the entire social security system. The 1967 social security ordinances governing the *caisses d'assurance maladie* (sickness funds) require them to assure a financial equilibrium of accounts. In case of deficit, they are empowered either to raise dues contributions or to reduce benefits expenditures. Such measures are subject to ratification by government decree. Further, if the funds do not ensure financial equilibrium, the government is authorized to take appropriate measures in place of the funds, superseding them entirely. Given the inevitably political nature of questions regarding social security contributions and benefits, it is clear that while the *caisses* administer social security on a daily basis, the real decision-making power lies with the government, including the Finance Ministry. Thus, while on paper the *caisses* are independent quasi-public bodies, in fact they are highly dependent on the government and the administration.

Consequences for Organized Medicine's Political Activities

The pattern of consultation, cooperation and contestation (characterized by a strong state and weak medical associations) affects a series of specific political activities. The more policy substance that is negotiated and/or decided at an administrative phase, the less remains to bargain over at a subsequent legislative phase. The French system is heavily weighted to administrative consultation; legislative strategies are consequently less important. In the American system, by contrast, consultation often occurs as legislation is being considered and more importance is attached to the legislative process. Consequently, the legislative strategies adopted – hand in hand with consultation – frequently change outcomes.

In general, the state initiates more contacts in France and *creates* more interests. Consultation is often part of a formal strategy by the French state to control interest sectors. Consultation also often serves as a symbolic benefit which administrators hope will forestall interest-group opposition, particularly protest and direct action which are common in France. Threatened or actual disturbances are a powerful influence on the administration to preserve at least the formalities of consultation. Finally, the state designates who is to be consulted, thus exercising formidable control over access. For the 1985 *convention* negotiations. Georgina Dufoix, Minister of Social Affairs and National Solidarity, *designated* both major medical confederations (the CSMF and the FMF) as representative of the profession and *conferred upon them* the sole right to negotiate with the *caisses d'assurance maladie* or sickness funds (*Le Médecin de France*, 29 November 1984: 18).

Organizational particularism in most interest sectors contributes to the lack of legitimacy of interest groups in state-dominated French society. It is difficult convincingly to claim representativeness for an interest when your group is not the only one making the claim and when many claims are coloured ideologically. Suleiman (1974: 337–40) notes that directors commonly distinguish between legitimate and illegitimate interests they must deal with. For the state administrators, lobbies and *groupes de pression* represent a private interest within an interest sector. These groups are not *sérieux*, an important concept to the French (Wylie 1957). Administrators prefer 'professional organizations', and contacts with them are considered valuable because these groups are *sérieux*, meaning reasonable, sincere and able to be counted upon: in short, 'responsible'. One director in Suleiman's study explained the distinction (1974: 338): 'An interest group – that is, a lobby – is one that defends its specific interest. A professional organization is one that defends not a private interest but a group [sectoral] interest.' Another director noted: 'An interest group or a pressure group has very limited interests, whereas professional organizations represent the interests of a whole profession.' Groups which are *sérieux* seek the public interest, not the private. The state determines who is *sérieux* and therefore a legitimate partner in the search for the public interest.

In negotiations with sickness funds, physicians manage to present a certain cohesiveness because fee negotiations are a politically neutral economic issue – neutral for physicians in the sense that all are affected similarly. Even in these cases, given the array of opposing interests and the structure of fee negotiating, physicians lose a great deal. They are not represented in the sickness funds, where for economic reasons management, workers and the state are united against raising fees. But even negotiating fees divides physicians and has highlighted their organizational particularism. The FMF alone signed the *conventions* of 1976 and 1980 which set fees for all private practitioners. Only recently have 25 years of bad blood between the CSMF and the FMF been superseded by a greater spirit of cooperation.

Further, it is the state that determines its own criteria for representativity. They are set out in article L261 of the Social Security Code and include the organization's number of years in existence, financial independence, membership size, and participation in the resistance during World War II. The general character of these criteria clearly allows the state wide latitude in designating which groups are worthy – or useful – interlocutors. For the 1985 *convention* negotiations, the administration received dossiers from seven medical associations, each claiming representativity and each seeking the conferral of bargaining powers. In the end, the Ministry of Social Affairs and National Solidarity designated the CSMF and the FMF – the two largest candidates – as the sole associations representative of the entire medical profession and thus the profession's sole negotiators for the 1985 *convention*.

In the United States, backers of controversial legislation generally adopt a strategy which looks to the gradual accretion of support (Marmor 1973: 80). The equivalent process in France looks very different. French bureaucrats or political appointees to the administration decide to press issues, with or without interest-group pressure. They may form an intraministerial committee for preliminary consideration. When the minister approves, the initiator contacts other ministries. Informal bargaining may lead quickly to a final version which could then be adopted by the Conseil des Ministres or approved by it for submission to the Assembly, where the government may use various tactics to secure passage easily. Sometimes an interministerial committee studies issues formally in order to resolve differences. The formation of such a committee may suggest the controversial nature of the issue at hand. Throughout the process, the finance ministry holds a pre-eminent position. Outside groups, including legislators, are seldom consulted at the outset but rather at the close of deliberations; they are included in negotiations in order to secure their support and to legitimate decisions already made (Mény 1985). The most important policy-making sphere is the administration, because the executive (the prime minister or the president) has great control over outcomes in the administrative and legislative arenas.

Electoral activities assume little importance for French physicians, especially regarding financial contributions, which are virtually absent. French medical associations' electoral activities are limited to two areas: information and in-kind support. The first is most prevalent and is aimed at informing members of the positions of different political parties at the national level and of specific candidates at the local level. To this end, associations at all levels examine parties' platforms and question candidates. The medical press – serving one of its most important functions – reports the results of these investigations. While associations usually take no official positions during an election, nor does the press generally take sides, members know which parties and candidates the associations and the press favour because of the positions that are endorsed. Of course, those associations identified with a particular ideology systematically endorse a specific political party.

While French medical associations seek to mobilize members' support for those candidates and parties which share the association's positions, no association contributes financially to any campaign. Without exception, no association has sufficiently secure or extensive financial resources to do so. Nevertheless, in-kind support is sometimes donated, usually from a local medical association to the campaign of a local doctor in politics. In-kind support takes the usual forms of stuffing envelopes, making calls and organizing meetings.

French medical associations' electoral activities are relatively unimportant because the French parliament is less influential in decision-making than the government and the administration. Further, the weak, divided French medical profession has few resources to devote to such activities.

Direct action is common in France. Even such supposedly pacific groups as physicians or hospital interns are quite willing to forgo traditional political channels in favour of boycotts, demonstrations and strikes. The use of strikes in particular, despite their questionable utility, indicates the highly reactive posture that the French state forces upon medical associations. In the United States, for example, strikes and other direct action are rare, because the medical profession could always exploit the dispersed structure of the American state.

Paradoxically, the prevalence of direct action in French politics and the frequency of violence that attends it attest to an important vulnerability of the French state. Dealing high-handedly with opponents cuts them off from normal avenues of negotiation and thereby forces them into direct action. In the tactical advantages that make the French state a strong countervailing force to interest groups lie also the seeds of that state's weakness.

Conclusion

While French physicians are united in their concern for professional privilege, particularism governs their organizing, thus weakening the profession in the face of state initiatives. Further, state initiatives in France are comprehensive, coherently connected and sustained. This strength comes from the state's concentration of power in a Colbert–Rousseauian distribution of political authority and from the tactical advantages which enable the state to make practical use of its theoretical power. The French state's strength combined with the medical profession's weakness led to a series of reforms throughout the post-war period which reduced the independence and power of French physicians. Hospital reforms, for example, were introduced in 1958, 1967 and 1969 under the Gaullists and in 1983 under the Socialists. Sweeping reform of liberal private practice medicine was undertaken in 1960. The freezing of physicians' fees through the social security system is undertaken regularly. The French state pursues more specific goals in structuring the role of the medical profession in the distribution of health care services and pursues these goals effectively. Each time, in the end, organized medicine's influence has been diminished.

Note

I wish to thank James W. Björkman, Henry W. Ehrmann, Giorgio Freddi, Arend Lijphart and Frank L. Wilson for their critical advice during the preparation of this chapter, as well as the French government for the privilege of serving as a Chateaubriand Fellow in 1985–6. The research reported here was undertaken during that period. All translations from French are mine; unattributed quotations are taken from personal interviews.

7

Hospital Planners and Medical Professionals in the Federal Republic of Germany

Christa Altenstetter

Power, authority, influence and control are ubiquitous phenomena (Dahl 1984). Scholars have studied them throughout the centuries, drawing on various theoretical approaches and reaching different conclusions (Friedrich 1963; Dahl 1961; Mills 1956; Lowi 1974; Marx and Engels 1969). Yet, in health, one standard repertoire has it that power, influence and control over strategic resources are concentrated in the professional sector, the bureaucratic sector and/or the industrial-pharmaceutical sector.

In the German context two major camps are said to be playing the leading roles and to have largely structured the discussions of health and hospital policy in the past (Naschold 1976). A conservative medical-industrial complex includes the conservative parties, medical corporate lobby groups and large sectors of the pharmaceutical industry. The social-bureaucratic complex consists of carriers of social insurance programmes, large segments of the trade unions and social democratic parties. On an abstract level and as macropolitical theory this suggestion is appealing, but as theory explaining the development and implementation of individual programmes (Rose 1984a, 1984b; Ashford 1978b; Altenstetter 1986b) it is speculative.

Federally structured political systems, and those where historically *Selbstverwaltungseinrichtungen* (self-governing and autonomous corporativist organizations) have carried out important national mandates, experience more scattered control over resources than do non-federal systems and/or those where a national health service serves as focal point of national policy. The political authority to decide on national policy, instruments and strategies is typically divided among several levels of government and between the governmental sectors and the corporativist organizations. The sheer number of consultations and decisions often hinders speedy decision-making and the adoption of optimal policy solutions (Scharpf et al. 1978; Scharpf 1985). Administrative and/or contractual responsibilities is even further dispersed at *Land* level. The point that needs stressing is that each level may control some resources (that is, political authority, finances, organizational resources, service providers, and information) necessary for one programme but typically not all.

The locus of power shifts from programme to programme, and so the question of who controls what, when, and under what circumstances is blurred. Consequently, the question of which level of government or which *Selbstverwaltung* is responsible for what can never be answered definitely for all programmes. The obstacles arising from dispersed control and multiple centres of authority and influence are nowhere more evident than in recent (largely unsuccessful) attempts at health planning, health promotion, the local coordination of health and social services (Hegner 1983, 1985a, 1985b) and the development of a coherent policy for the elderly (Merschbrock-Bäuerle et al. 1985). Who controls resources allocation at the boundaries of primary medical and health care and social services is even more complex to answer globally (Schwefel 1985; Koenen and Riedmüller 1982; Bonß and Riedmüller 1982; Badura and von Ferber 1981, 1983; Kickbusch and Trojan 1981; Waller 1985; Leibfried and Tennstedt 1985; Müller and Wasem 1984; Krüger and Pankoke 1985; Labisch 1985; Riedmüller 1980).

How corporatism has been functioning in highly diverse political and socio-cultural environments has been the subject of many comparative studies (Lehmbruch and Schmitter 1982; Schmitter and Lehmbruch 1979). While such analyses are eminently pertinent, specific historical differences have unfortunately been sacrificed in favour of a desire to conceptualize at a high level of abstraction and to discover converging developments across modern industrial nations. Case studies are therefore few in number. The health and medical care field, however, deserves special attention because the number and variety of professional and other interest groups far exceeds those in other economic sectors. Groups range from the corporately organized and mandatory medical, dental and pharmaceutical professional organizations, through an array of mostly voluntary groups of nurses, chiropractors, auxiliaries, orthopaedic shoemakers and self-help groups, to numerous professional associations of academic medicine and medical specialties and sub-specialties (Schulenburg 1984).

By way of summary, within-sector variations of patterns of decision-making, influence and control in one and the same policy sector, the same country, and the same constitutional federal framework are significant. They fundamentally challenge monocausal explanations. This descriptive analysis focuses on the Hospital

Financing Act of 1972 (KHG) and its implementation from 1972 to 1984 by drawing on fieldwork in two German *Länder* (Altenstetter 1980, 1982, 1985a, 1985b, 1985c, 1986a) and occasionally on information concerning all eleven *Länder*. The aim is to discover who are the prime actors, who controls the strategic resources, and who occupies the strategic positions. The term 'strategic' is used in a historical-political rather than a behavioural sense of 'strategic linkage choice' (Friend and Noad 1977). The analysis begins with a brief review of the role of the *Länder* in hospital policy which intersects with the statutory health insurance programme (GKV). It then outlines the major goals and instruments mandated by the Hospital Financing Act of 1972. Next, it addresses how national hospital policy is managed in circumstances of fragmented constitutional and political authority and responsibilities. Hospital need planning and hospital reimbursement are then discussed for Bavaria and North Rhine Westphalia (NRW), while a final section focuses on medical professionals and the part they play in these processes.

The Role of the *Länder*

The Basic Law of 1949 assigns the *Länder* a most powerful and prominent role in hospital and health matters. In 1969 a constitutional amendment opened the way to joint federal/*Land* financing (*Mischfinanzierung*) of medical schools in 1971, and short-term hospitals in 1972. Even under joint financing from 1972 to 1984 the *Länder* have asserted their interests. They own and run university hospitals. They fund the payroll of hospital workers and professional staff in medical schools. They enforce federal requirements for accreditation, licensing and qualification of staff and facilities. They supervise medical education and research. Most importantly, they remain responsible for the effective and efficient allocation and distribution of resources and medical capacities through hospital need planning and hospital payment policy. Moreover, the *Länder* play an important role in most areas pertaining to nursing homes, public assistance or social aid, social welfare services, and social work.

Policy Context and Background

GKV goals and programmatic hospital objectives are highly interdependent and, hence, require a brief background. GKV is a 100-year-old entitlement programme insuring about 10 percent of the population in 1883 and more than 90 percent in 1985. It provides fairly comprehensive coverage for all risks of chronic or temporary illness and physical, mental, or emotional disability as well as income protection. It provides for all diagnostic and therapeutic services which are necessary and medically feasible, independent of whether they are delivered in offices or hospitals. Today GKV is an all-inclusive health protection and income maintenance programme.

GKV is unique in Europe even when compared with other countries which have moved towards a national health service. The administration of GKV rests on an organizational model – *Selbstver-waltung* – formally independent of public sector administration (von Ferber 1978, 1985; Tennstedt 1977; Mayntz et al. 1982; Wuster 1985; Neubauer 1985). By relying on about 950 insurance funds each controlled by an equal number of employees' and employers' representatives, and another 350 funds which are organized and controlled differently, the administration of GKV is highly de-centralized and pluralistic.

The funds are organized by geographical district, occupation, or enterprise. They pay the bulk of all medical, dental, pharmaceutical and hospital bills in Germany, which amounted to about 9.3 percent of GNP in 1983. Moreover, they plan crucial intervening, facilitating and supporting roles in the operations of hospital programmes, some programmes of the German social security system, and labour market programmes, to mention just a few. About 95 percent of a fund's income derives from contributions calculated as a percentage of wages and salaries based on a national income ceiling. A fund sets the actual percentage as a function of (1) local salary and wage developments and (2) the expenditures of the fund. To balance the books, funds have set different rates ranging from 6.5 percent to 14.8 percent in 1983 (Bundesminister für Arbeit und Sozialordnung 1985: T11).

Despite their important role as implementing agencies, they have no authority to decide for whom, under what conditions, and for what services they spend their resources. Nor do they influence the amounts that they pay for medical and dental services or drug bills per patient. These issues are decided by national policy and/or joint contractual agreements negotiated between national and regional associations of insurance carriers and organized physicians' interest (Neubauer and Rebscher 1984). Or, they result directly from hospital need planning and the high cost of new hospitals. Local funds have retained some influence over the setting of hospital rates (which constitute about 32 percent of total GKV expenditures).

According to the health insurance code (section 184 Abs. 2 RVO), members of a fund are supposed to go to the nearest and most adequate hospital. If they choose, for example, a university clinic which is more expensive, they are supposed to pay the difference. But practice differs considerably from the law. Physicians do not apply strict interpretations when admitting patients, and nor do sickness funds enforce these rules. Hospitalization of over 90 percent of Germans is governed by *Krankenhausverträge* contracted between hospitals and sickness funds which guarantee to pay for hospitalization. Hospitalization of the remaining Germans is typically governed by private contracts. At the same time, hospital laws secure the delivery of hospital services to any patient independent of financial means or social status (Behrends 1983).

Over time *Selbstverwaltung* has become subject to the growing influence of federal and *Land* legislation, regulations, and the joint agreements of corporativist organizational elites of physicians and sickness funds. Because of a time-honoured 'mobilization of biases' and institutionalized values and preferences (Schattschneider 1960), it has also become rigid, immobile, and largely closed to innovation.

The Hospital Financing Act of 1972

Generally, the Hospital Financing Act of 1972 (KHG) pursued three goals:

1 To provide hospitals with a viable economic base
2 To develop a regionalized hospital care system by distributing facilities, beds, services, and medical technological hardware in all regions and communities
3 To set reasonable user charges that could be financed by the public health insurance scheme (NHI).

The process of administering and developing guidelines for the implementation of the Act has led to the creation of fairly autonomous subprogrammes involved either with hospital care finance or with planning and finance of capital investments.

One of these subprogrammes (designed to achieve the third goal in the above list), the Federal Regulation on User Charges (BPflV), specified how GKV would finance recurrent expenditures, namely wages and maintenance in hospitals. The regulation reinforced the principles that costs should be based on occupancy per bed per day, and that rates should cover costs, by requiring effectiveness, efficiency and economic management without clearly defining what these concepts were to mean operationally. To provide some assistance, the federal regulation introduced two policy instruments. The first was a complex hospital accounting form (*Selbstkostenblatt*, over 30 pages in comparison to about four pages previously) formally establishing a commercial budgeting and accounting system and abolishing the 200-year-old Prussian cameral system. Its intended purpose was to rationalize hospital rate setting so that in-depth, mainly input-related information on hospital expenditures might be generated (Altenstetter 1986a).

Secondly, final rates were to be set in direct negotiations between hospitals and sickness funds. Federal and *Land* regulations provided detailed specifications on how this task was to be carried out. This federal strategy was highly interventionist and was only the first of a series of regulations that would considerably interfere with hospital autonomy.

Another subprogramme of the Act of 1972 (to achieve the first and second goals in the above list, and restricted to short-term hospitals) regulated how hospital construction, renovation and investments in technological hardware should be financed. The subprogramme also regulated the distribution of hospitals, technological hardware and beds according to a certificate-of-need process (Brown 1983). Although federally initiated, this programme was intended mainly to be administered at *Land* level. The Act specified minimum objectives of hospital need planning and stipulated the conditions under which this was to be carried out. The Act prescribed the following:

1 A minimum size of hospitals over 100 beds
2 The development of hospitals with different care levels
3 The identification of need depending on the type of funding
4 The annual review of three policy instruments, namely hospital need plans, multiyear hospital programmes, and annual construction programmes
5 The participation of hospital associations, third-party payers and other groups.

These regulatory details further curtailed the budgetary and organizational autonomy of hospitals and negatively affected third-party payers. They had to pay for whatever additional operating costs resulted from hospital need planning. Their participation in the planning process could not compensate for this lack of influence.

These goals – a viable economic base, a regionalized hospital care system and reasonable user charges – could be obtained only in a growing economy. As resources became more limited during and after the 1973 oil crisis, demands for corrective measures were increasingly heard. A Cost Containment Act of 1977 (Krankenversicherungs-Kostendämpfungsgesetz: KVKG) imposed certain restrictions on private medical and dental providers, members of GKV and on the pharmaceutical industry but excluded the hospital sector. The Hospital Cost Containment Act (Krankenhaus-Kostendämpfungsgesetz: KHKG) of 1981 sought cost controlling measures and requested that future costs resulting from hospital need planning and capital-intensive biomedical technology (Krebs and John 1985) be considered in planning and rate setting. The Krankenhaus-Neuordnungsgesetz (KHNG) became effective on 1 January 1985, and abolished joint federal/*Land* financing of capital investments and technological hardware. The KHNG restored the status quo ante and allowed the *Länder* to prove their claims that they can do a better job of setting priorities to meet current and future needs. The KHNG intends to strengthen the role of individual hospitals and sickness funds and *Selbstverwaltung*.

A new Federal Regulation on User Charges became effective on 1 January 1986 (BPflV). It dramatically altered the existing method of reimbursing hospitals by introducing a so-called flexible and prospective budget to be calculated on the basis of anticipated occupancy rates in the forthcoming year (Zimmer 1985). Hospitals and sickness funds must agree on the items or rates which make up the budget. If they fail to agree, a neutral and non-governmental arbitration office is called upon to fix them. Special rates for severe and costly diseases such as cancer, renal dialysis, and thorax surgery have always been accepted. The new regulation requests that additional rate categories be developed for lithotripsy and other disease categories. In the era of neo-conservatism supply-side health economists and politicians (*WSI Mitteilungen* 1985) toy with the idea of moving toward a DRG-based reimbursement scheme (Simborg 1981; Wennberg et al. 1984; May and Wasserman 1985), although the organizational, structural and policy conditions as well as the information basis vary highly from those prevailing in the United States. Cost containment in the future? Hardly.

The 'reform act of the century', as it was hailed in 1972, did not last a decade; nor did it produce the expected results. It was instead held responsible for accelerated rates of inflation. Political pressures to alter the existing methods of resource allocation, planning and financing and to upgrade the participation of insurance carriers and hospitals in planning have, however, been partially successful.

Problems of Coordinating National Hospital Policy

How can national hospital policy be coordinated when lines of authority and responsibility for hospital policy are unclear and/or fragmented? Germany tried to manage by using two approaches. The first was the creation of a federal/*Land* coordinating committee mostly composed of members of the various ministries in Bonn and the *Länder*. Its responsibility was to ensure that the *Länder*, which were in full constitutional and political control of these issues, would approach long-term investments, their distribution and location in similar ways. A subcommittee was to coordinate hospital payment policies and to harmonize those decisions in which they retained some discretion. Unlike the planning programme, the federal government retained considerable control over the formulation of reimbursement policy.

Hospitals and third-party payers complained that the federal/ *Land* committees were bureaucratically dominated and excluded those mostly affected by planning decisions. In lobbying for a change in legislation, they supported different positions. Sickness funds requested independent arbitration, whereas hospitals required more protection by the state. The KHNG now requires the establishment of arbitration offices in each *Land*.

A second mechanism exists for coordinating policy. The KVKG of 1977 set up a national 60-member council (Konzertierte Aktion) which would recommend admissible rates of increases related to the revenues of GKV (Siebig 1981; Wiesenthal 1981). The slowing down of the inflation rate in health expenditures can hardly be assigned to the effectiveness of the council alone (contrary to Schulenburg 1983; Stone 1980; Glaser 1983). As a national steering instrument to influence the health and hospital sector its performance has been at best modest. Its recommendations largely reflect either prior agreements between the major parties concerned, symbolic gestures, or consensus on unimportant issues. The *Länder* have successfully kept the hospital sector outside this council's purview, and it is unlikely that in the near future they will abdicate their new responsibilities and accept central recommendations, unless these coincide with their own preferences.

Regional initiatives of corporativist organizations of RVO funds and physicians in Bavaria, Hesse, Lower Saxony and Berlin provide evidence that the authority of the council is fundamentally challenged, although the biannual rituals, promises and exhortations continue. By providing collective incentives to office-based physicians, the physicians were expected to take full advantage of them and thereby help to shift resources from the hospital sector to the non-hospital sector. Of these regional initiatives the so-called Bavarian Contract is the most interesting and far-reaching (Schwefel et al. 1986b). Satzinger (1986a, 1986b) describes the Bayern-Vertrag as being 'anti-centralist' and 'anti-dirigist' and challenging the Bonn government of 1979 and the council. The latter have both been seeking nationally uniform solutions for each care subsector separately. Other political groups have challenged the federal government and the council, but they are too numerous to be included here. Indeed, managing policy interdependencies in health and hospital care across governmental levels, between governmental and non-governmental institutions and through *Selbstverwaltungen* at the national and regional levels has been difficult in the past.

Hospital Need Planning in Bavaria and North Rhine Westphalia 1972–84

Within broad federal goals, the *Länder* are responsible for financing hospital investments, technological hardware and hospital need planning (Altenstetter 1985a, 1985b, 1985c). Enabling *Land* legislation – being amended presently – states broad planning goals. With the exception of Bremen, Hamburg, Saarland, and Schleswig-Holstein, all *Länder* have developed a hospital need plan. However, no plan distinguishes between primary and secondary needs, that is, between need for diagnostic and therapeutic services, and need for beds, medical technology and quality. Apart from Hesse and Lower Saxony, all *Länder* set up comprehensive procedures and participatory mechanisms, including the designation of geographical or administrative areas as planning areas (Schön et al. 1978).

Political and administrative background
Hospital need planning has differed considerably across *Länder* because of different circumstances and conditions in the delivery of care in each *Land*; the particular status of hospital need planning when the KHG was enacted; different circumstances in the extent of divided authority and responsibilities of *Land* offices and bureaux; and considerable differences in administrative organization and political-administrative culture. The *Länder* also set the amount which the cities and counties contribute to the programme. The local shares differ from *Land* to *Land*. For example, NRW settled for a local share of 20 percent of total expenditures, the remaining 80 percent being paid for by the *Land*. Bavarian municipalities and counties pay the highest share in Germany, namely half of all capital expenditures.

In most *Länder* the same ministerial/bureaucratic, territorial and functional interests which played leading roles in hospital planning prior to 1972 were recognized relevant policy actors after 1972. Responsibilities of ministries were reorganized. Central ministries became fully responsible for this programme. The rationale for centralizing decision-making was standardized medical, technical, technological and economic as well as architectural criteria in each *Land*. Standardization naturally increases the power and authority of those who define its meaning.

The Ministry of Labour, Health and Social Affairs (MAGS) in

NRW and the Ministry of Labour and Social Order (StMAS) in Bavaria were in no way bashful about concentrating responsibilities and using their newly gained power, influence and control. Since 1972 StMAS in Bavaria has been the leading ministry responsible for the hospital need plan and the administration of the KHG. All decisions on individual projects and overall planning, however, require the approval of the Ministry of Finance which controls all resources allocation. It is also responsible for the grants-in-aid programme by which the communities contribute to the capital investment programme. Planning also requires impact statements by the Ministries of the Environment and of Urban Development. Decisions on university hospitals have to be coordinated with the Ministry of Culture and Education. Finally, decision-making frequently involves the Ministry of the Interior responsible for local government affairs. Indeed, inter- and intraministerial rivalries and shared responsibilities have not facilitated consensus.

The nearly omnipotent position of MAGS in relation to other ministries, regional offices, hospitals, funds and local governments in NRW rested on three resources which it controlled. First, MAGS manoeuvred early to obtain full control of a global hospital budget which it administered independently after approval of the Ministry of Finance had been obtained, subject only to the provisions that guide the use of public funds. Secondly, MAGS was also at an advantage because it generated, processed and interpreted in-house an array of data, statistics and surveys which were not available elsewhere. The control over the production and use of its own information gave the ministry unequalled power which it used for its own strategies. Thirdly, it obtained control over all responsibilities relating to medical-technological matters from the Ministry of the Interior. It also gained control over construction matters from the previously existing Ministry of Construction in 1971. In other words, all administrative responsibilities and controls over planning, financing, medical-technological and construction matters were concentrated in MAGS.

MAGS did not control one important hospital sector either politically or administratively, namely medical schools and teaching hospitals owned by the *Land* and subject to the Ministry of Science and Technology. MAGS intended to remove all primary care services from the expensive university hospitals and to transfer them to primary care hospitals. These plans encountered the fierce opposition of Science and Technology and its political allies. Moreover, high hospital rates in university and teaching hospitals were another serious bone of contention between the two ministries and third-party payers aligned with MAGS. Finally, both ministries and, above all, non-university and teaching hospitals differed with one another concerning realistic assumptions of average occupancy and utilization rates in university and teaching hospitals. But eventually MAGS in alliance with its own political supporters prevailed upon the Ministry of Science and Technology and university and teaching hospitals.

*Centralism versus regionalism in hospital need planning:
bread and circuses*

Bavaria's approach to hospital need planning is centralist and pragmatic. Bavaria, in tune with its tradition of political and bureaucratic centralism, chose to establish a central planning committee which has advisory responsibilities and reports to MAGS. It developed its first and only hospital need plan in 1974 which has been amended twelve times since then. Its members are the core ministries and all relevant health and hospital groups in Bavaria. Pragmatism suggests that the determinants used in planning be reviewed annually, such as the number of beds allotted to medical specialties and subspecialties in hospitals, population, occupancy rates, length of stay and the like.

The most dramatic changes in the hospital sector occurred between 1972 and 1975. Numerous hospitals were approved conditionally and/or temporarily. Of over 500 hospitals some 200 received a temporary proviso. Of 402 fully approved hospitals in 1980, 110 still retained a few restrictions. As a result of legal problems and political pressures, all provisos were dropped entirely by 1980. In 1978 the revised plan redefined a total of 56 hospitals previously classified as complementary to the regular hospitals. Hospitals with an average occupancy rate below 80 percent during the previous three years and those with an average length of stay of over twenty days were ordered to reduce bed capacities. In 1981 and 1982 new medical subspecialties were approved for purposes of public funding. Following the KHKG of 1981 the plan stressed cost containment, the need for cooperation, the joint use of expensive medical-technological hardware by hospitals and their distribution in economically run hospital units. In balancing these issues Bavaria seems to be guided by considerations that hospital policy should offer investment and employment opportunities as well as diagnostic and therapeutic services and care.

The original hospital need plan reflected planners' high expectations about the feasibility of inter- and intrasectoral policy and service coordination. The plan is in three parts. Part I states general and specific principles, the scope of planning and guidelines. Part II lists all hospitals needed in each of seven hospital care areas whose boundaries are coterminous with those of the seven administrative districts. Hospitals are classified according to site, ownership and number of approved beds, care levels and medical specialties. Finally, Part II lists those projects which are approved for public funding in a particular year. These provisions remain valid.

Part III survived publication only a few years. It outlined long-term goals and regional objectives, of which some were realized by incremental measures, but outside the hospital need plan and contrary to the planners' intention. Why? Integrative planning requires the cooperation and coordination of hospital and social policy across macro-policy domains and the coordination of services across medical, social and health service sectors. But party politicians in the *Land* and local communities had as many diverse views about the scope and purpose of coordination as had representatives from different medical specialties and other professions. Bureaucratic segments in different ministries and umbrella associations of sickness funds, physicians, hospitals and public and private charities carefully protected their respective turf.

Failing to reach a consensus, policy actors since 1980 have stressed sectoral programmes. Centres serve renal dialysis patients, patients requiring therapeutic radiology, radiation victims, and heart and stroke patients. Ambulance and emergency services were improved and trauma centres were financed. Bavaria's experiences in encountering impediments – political, bureaucratic, professional and organizational – to the coordination of policy and services in a planning document which would be binding on all health actors were by no means unique, nor are the problems fully solved. Other *Länder* confronted similar obstacles and moved, therefore, in the same direction of largely supporting incremental steps and sectoral programmes.

NRW opted for a decentralized strategy and heard the policy actors, prescribed by the KHG and *Land* law, at regional meetings in each of its sixteen hospital planning regions. The option in favour of a relatively large circle of political groups, instead of a few elite spokespersons in Bavaria, is consonant with the social-political milieu and administrative traditions and practices. Governments in NRW have oscillated between a right and a centre-left orientation. Until 1966 the government was either Conservative or a Conservative-Liberal coalition. A Social-Liberal coalition was in power between 1966 and 1980, and a Social-Democratic government has been in power since then. A decentralized approach can accommodate deep-seated regional differences between the two territorial parts, Rhineland and Westphalia, and their respective hospital interests. In contrast, a Conservative government has been in power uninterruptedly in Bavaria since 1947.

MAGS and third-party payers were in agreement about the general planning strategy that predated 1972, but they sharply differed with the hospital association and other groups on two matters which were crucial because NRW had developed binding, medium-term hospital need plans instead of annual reviews. Three hospital need plans have been operative since 1974. Hospital planners found it very difficult to predict population changes accurately, and they were usually wrong. In 1977 and 1978 when the third plan was prepared, an initial dispute concerned the question of whether average *Land* values on frequency and length of stay should be applied when corresponding values in particular regions diverged from this average. The second disagreement concerned proper population forecasts. MAGS relied on aggregate population forecasts, while the cities and counties typically used disaggregated population data broken down by smaller geographical units and more favourable to them.

Many discussions in municipal and county committees preceded the regional meetings. In addition, individual hospitals had meetings with their respective umbrella association, the hospital association, and sometimes the local departments of health. The purpose of these meetings was to develop and present to MAGS a local or regional consensus which forced heterogeneous political and hospital interests in particular regions to sort out their differences and come up with a unified vision of the delivery of hospital services in a region. There were individual losers and winners. But collectively they could hardly match the power of MAGS. The local advisory hospital councils, mandated by law in 1975, were excluded from the regional meetings, but they gave the appearance of grassroots participation. Because the law failed to define exactly what their responsibilities were to be, they had little identity. Overlapping membership in the local health and social committees and the hospital council somewhat counterbalanced this powerlessness, and eventually they gained some influence.

MAGS prepared and distributed an impressive amount of information about all hospital infrastructures and services in each region and used by far the most comprehensive data and sophisticated methods (Schön et al. 1978). Judging by the results (Bundesminister für Arbeit und Sozialordnung 1985), however, NRW hardly fares better than the remaining *Länder* which were all guided primarily by considerations of the availability or non-availability of resources rather than of the need for services (Altenstetter 1985a: 109–60).

What were the real objectives of these meetings? They are of four kinds. First, regional meetings are more practical, so MAGS argued, than individual meetings with each of the more than 600 hospitals in North Rhine Westphalia. But numerous meetings with individual hospital and medical representatives in the ministry preceded and followed the regional meetings. Secondly, the government and MAGS intended to display administrative and political authority in all regions which require problem-solving arrangements that simultaneously express territorial interests. Thirdly, regional meetings were spectacular and offered opportunities to stage impressive political shows and to demonstrate how sensitive government planners were to the grassroots. In touring the country in a mobile bus rather than bringing policy actors to the capital, as Bavaria did, the ministerial bureaucracy of MAGS and other ministries established close contacts with regional and local constituencies. No doubt these efforts left their political imprint. Finally, regional meetings were intended to legitimize decisions which MAGS had already reached or was going to reach, and to reduce conflicts. Participants could give warning signals that MAGS should expect considerable opposition to its proposals before the final hospital plan would be finalized and approved by parliament. On the other hand MAGS was requested to present and publicly justify the reasons for its decisions on care levels, bed reductions, closure, temporary acceptance and the like.

Were the differences between the two *Länder* merely those of form and style, or were there, in addition, differences in accountability over the content and substance of planning decisions (Björkman and Altenstetter 1979)? The evidence suggests that the differences are largely those of form and political style. In both *Länder* the central ministries have controlled decision-making. Hospitals were not treated as independent voices. Instead, they had to work through, and rely on, *Land* spokespersons in Bavaria and regional spokespersons in NRW. The central planning committee and the regional meetings were advisory bodies only. Finally, in both *Länder* no change in governmental or ministerial leadership occurred as a result of a 'crisis' in hospital finance and hospital need planning.

Regional offices
Despite political differences, the administrative organization and the pattern of regional and central communication is fairly similar. Four bureaux deal with either medical-technological issues and aspects of technological hardware, construction, investment funds and hospital rates. But individually and collectively they could in no

way use the new and comprehensive responsibilities to their own political advantage. The regional offices received comprehensive sets of supporting documents which they transmitted from ministry to hospitals and vice versa. In short, they were obedient civil servants executing central decisions. Although regional offices were to 'supervise', 'control', 'consider special circumstances' and 'provide medical-technological, technical, and architectural and financial expertise', their decisions were reviewed again by a central and analogous set of experts who had the final word.

Hospital Reimbursement Policy

The BPflV of 1974 meticulously outlined extensive federal powers and reinforced federal policy-making authority over hospital payment policies (Altenstetter 1982). The new BPflV continues this pattern. Within this framework, the *Länder* retained considerable leeway and discretion which officials used flexibly and by trial and error. The differences in administrative policy were a function not simply of differences in *Land* law and administrative routines but also of the different political interpretations of what the primary goals and objectives of federal hospital policy were supposed to be. Although 'no single goal was to be overrated to the detriment of one party' (Oetzel 1981: 147), ministries and officials were known to be partisan towards either the hospitals or the sickness funds. For some the control of hospital costs was said to be of high priority; for others the goal was the provision of quality services independent of the costs required to provide them.

Regional price offices were to evaluate the economic and medical behaviour of hospitals and to reconcile the three contradictory goals inherent in the federal legislation. Four major areas were to receive attention by the reviewers: salaries, services, management and maintenance. The categories are simple, and their crude measures hardly furnish significant indicators of efficiency, effectiveness and economic management; nor do they reveal significant aspects of medical services, nursing care, diagnosis, therapy and cure. As Thiemeyer's (1979, 1981) empirical analyses have shown, the new hospital accounting system in reality never replaced the old system of budgeting and accounting, incorporating elements of a cameral and a commercial accounting system. Additional complex changes were introduced in 1986. The coexistence of two entirely different principles created numerous problems in implementation (Altenstetter 1985a: 41–108). Hospital audits conducted under these circumstances can hardly be considered reviews of economic management, medical efficiency or effectiveness. In a political-administrative culture which stresses legal traditions, normativism and formalism they are more likely reviews of legal and procedural conformity.

These offices formally were to certify the charges for occupancy per bed per day. In some *Länder* these charges are set by the offices; in others they are directly negotiated between the sickness funds and hospitals and ratified by regional offices which had backup support from the ministry. The two parties were estimated to have reached agreements on rates in the first round in about 90 to 95 percent of all cases (Altenstetter 1982). Schnabel (1980) reported on a similar record in Baden-Württemberg – about 80 percent of all cases. Zimmer (1985: 759) reports that 97 percent of all negotiations between hospitals and sickness funds resulted in rates that were accepted as final in Bavaria. The remaining 3 percent were disputed in court.

The high frequency of agreements in the two *Länder* is also explained by the power of persuasion and subtle and/or overt threats which regional offices, supported by their respective ministries, have used. They have an advantage over hospitals and sickness funds by manoeuvring and manipulating each side, thus forcing them into an agreement. If the fund is not pleased with the proposed rate, the office could threaten that the final rate would be even higher. In turn, it could threaten a hospital to set fees at a rate lower than the hospital had requested.

The hospital associations and the associations of corporativist sickness funds (LdO) are the most important non-governmental actors in hospital rate setting, but they are not the only ones. By many standards of comparison the two parties are not equal partners (Altenstetter 1985a; Satzinger et al. 1984). In each *Land* the LdO is a homogeneous mandatory membership organization of general sickness funds (AOKs). Both have public law status. In contrast, hospital associations have no public law status. They are loose associations of membership organizations rather than of individual hospitals, and this prevents them from taking on a strong leadership role. About 70 percent of hospitals in Bavaria are owned by cities and counties. Cities and counties are members of separate municipal associations which compete with each other for influence in the policy-making process. Private voluntary hospitals – almost 20 percent – are members of their respective charitable associations which, in turn, are also members of the hospital associations. Private for-profit hospitals are organized separately in the Verband der Privatanstalten.

In NRW the hospital association is hampered even more than its counterpart in Bavaria. First, it faces the strong rivalry between hospital associations and working groups which exists in West-phalia. Secondly, there is an equally pronounced competition for influence and prestige among ten membership organizations reflect-ing heterogeneous hospital ownership, notably denominational ownership. Thirdly, conflicts between hospitals and sickness funds make life difficult. And, finally, hospital interests located in the two territories, North Rhine and Westphalia, require special consider-ation. Undoubtedly these political factors undermine any strong leadership of the hospital association *vis-à-vis* sickness funds, governments and ministries.

Medical Professionals

In 1967 Rohde spoke of a *terra incognita* of systematic analyses of the role of physicians and hospitals (Rohde 1967: 349–61). While most medical sociologists (such as Reimann and Reimann 1976; Siegrist 1978; Höflich 1984) confirm Freidson's (1975) findings on the dominance of the medical profession – its hierarchy, culture, autonomy, division of labour and the like – empirical studies are still missing. Little is known about the hospital medical profession and academic medicine and about how this hierarchy (medical director, chief physician, ward physician and/or assistant physician) has impacted on hospital need planning and rate setting. More can be said about the indirect influence of professional dominance, and about the widely shared consensus that medical progress should be made available to all patients independent of whether they pay through GKV, PHI or out of pocket.

Certainly physicians play a dominant role in hospitals, determin-ing length of stay, occupancy rates, admission and discharge, and diagnosing and treating single and multiple morbidity. By engaging in all these activities, they considerably determine hospital expendi-tures. Physicians are, therefore, publicly accused of cooperating with hospital administrators in order to increase cases by discharging patients over weekends and readmitting them on Monday, reassign-ing patients from one ward to another, and admitting patients in emergency cases or when they come directly to a hospital on their own rather than by referral – the normal mechanism under GKV. Much as this charge stirs up the health policy debate, it remains unsubstantiated (Potthoff and Leidl 1986).

In all *Länder* the hospital medical profession participated in hos-pital need planning in several ways. Bavaria's central planning committee included one medical representative of the Ärztekammer, and regional meetings in NRW included two representatives of corporativist medicine. In addition, local committees had medical representation. In negotiating user charges, the medical director of a hospital is typically a member of the hospital delegation. The staff in each ministry and the regional offices included several medically trained civil servants.

However, it is difficult to sort the power of bureaucratic hospital planners who control the money from the power of medical professionals who control the expertise and promise care and cure. To specify in individual cases whether and how professional dominance and preferences were brought to bear on decisions is next to impossible. Yet medical influence, power and considerations are present in federal laws, hospital plans and regulations concerning hospital reimbursement, the financing and distribution of technological hardware and medical capacities and facilities.

Hospitals are grouped according to the number and the functions of medical departments and available medical-technological capabilities. In determining groups the *Länder* were to take into account (1) the number of medical specialties or subfields headed by a full-time specialist, (2) the number of additional fully employed or licensed specialists in other subspecialties and who were not heads of departments, and (3) available facilities and technological skills and hardware. As previously mentioned, special rates for specialized treatment centres and special diseases have been possible since 1972. Now hospitals are required to keep records on diagnoses by specialty ward. From 1988 they have had to record age and duration of stay of patients.

As a rule, hospital physicians cannot treat out-patients. However, certain physicians retained a right to bill in-patients willing to pay extra for personal services rendered, and out-patients treated using the facilities of the hospital. The former are typically the holders of PHI (7.5 percent of the German population) and members of GKV who carry PHI, in addition to GKV (8.5 percent of the population), and a few who pay out of pocket. Physicians who have these privileges are typically medical directors at university hospitals and/or teaching hospitals. To use these facilities, they are required to pay 6 percent of revenues earned on this basis to the hospital. The national fee schedule which applies to office charges also applies here (Zacher 1985). Their remaining incomes are civil service salaries. Conflicts over these privileges exist not only with professional segments excluded from these rights, office physicians, and the bulk of the population, but also with PHI and hospitals. Rates charged for hospitalization of patients treated under these circumstances by the hospitals are 15 percent less than those charged to GKV.

There are numerous other links between hospital medicine and hospital need planning and reimbursement. In reassigning medical specialties and subspecialties within a hospital for purposes of public funding, hospital planners recognized medical progress in diagnosis and therapy, drug therapies and high-tech medicine, and processes internal to the medical profession such as increased subspecialization and functional differentiation. For purposes of public funding, planners in Bavaria recognized fifteen different medical specialties, and later eighteen. Planners in NRW recognized eighteen medical disciplines in 1968, nineteen in 1971 and twenty in 1980, and they recognized geriatric care and nuclear medicine as two separate specialties in allocating beds. Moreover, they subdivided internal medicine and surgery into additional medical subspecializations.

A comparison of the distribution of beds by disciplines between 1967 and 1985 in NRW gives some impression of the influence of academic medicine. In relative and proportional terms more beds are now allocated to emergency surgery, neurosurgery, orthopaedics, urology, internal medicine with subspecialties, gynaecology, geriatrics, radiology and psychiatry, including psychiatry for children and youth. These increases are directly associated with demographic and epidemiological developments and diagnostic and therapeutic progress in medical knowhow, as reductions of resources (in obstetrics, children's wards and tuberculosis) reflect declining birth rates and progress in treating tuberculosis. With one exception, however, changes over this period remained within a modest ±2 percent margin.

Other links exist between academic medicine and hospital need planning and rate setting. North Rhine Westphalia funds 59 teaching hospitals associated with her six medical schools, and Bavaria 31 teaching hospitals associated with her four medical schools. Although teaching hospitals and medical schools are formally included in the hospital need plan of each *Land* and the beds are 'counted' they are exempted from many restrictions placed on all other hospitals. Typically, their interests have taken precedence over the remaining hospitals.

By way of summary, hospital planners adjusted to medical progress and technological developments. Specialty fields and subfields have changed markedly during the last twenty years, largely as the result of professional segments competing for prestige and resources. Rapid diffusion of medical technology occurred mainly after 1980. In early 1985 a total of 2146 items of medical equipment qualified as large-scale biomedical devices (*medizinische Großgeräte*). Of these 1491 or 70 percent were in hospitals, the remaining 655 or 30 percent in doctors' offices (Bruckenberger 1985).

Concluding Comments

Within-sector variations of patterns of decision-making, authority, influence and control in one and the same policy sector, country, and constitutional framework are significant. Policy context and process analyses are indispensable tools.

A host of substantive compromises were necessary because of time-honoured institutional arrangements for policy-making on GKV, hospital infrastructure financing and hospital need planning as well as hospital rate setting. Compromises on substance have characterized both recent and long-term developments. In theory, systemic and institutional reforms could have allowed the emergence of single centres of authority, influence and control in hospital matters. For historical, constitutional and political reasons these were not forthcoming. Authority, influence and control over hospital resources remain divided and are scattered among governmental and non-governmental actors. Decisions are taken in multiple centres of control and influence such as legislatures, ministries, administrative offices, policy committees, corporativist organizations, umbrella associations, hospital and sickness funds as well as the courts.

While systematic studies on academic medicine and the hospital medical profession and their respective influence on hospital need planning are still lacking for Germany, there is no doubt that the two groups have played a significant role. Professional preferences and diagnostic and therapeutic practices have been respected by civil service hospital planners who supported medical progress. But it is difficult to sort out the power of bureaucratic hospital planners who control the purse from that of medical professionals who control medical expertise and decisions on care and cure. Both groups share similar values and perceptions about medicine and what is needed to practise it effectively and efficiently to the satisfaction of the public.

Constitutional assignment policies remained stable from 1972 to 1984. During this period the political authority of the *Länder* as the most influential actor group increased considerably with regard to the hospital need planning and investment programme but less in the hospital rate setting programme. *Festsetzung*, as the administrative process was called, has served as a formal mechanism, and hospitals and sickness funds have been the actual negotiators.

With the enactment of KHNG and BPflV in 1985 and 1986, respectively, the era of joint federal/*Land* policy-making characteristic of the period from 1972 to 1985 legally came to an end. It has been replaced by decentralized decision-making and problem-solving by the *Länder* and, above all, hospital and sickness funds. If these intentions are to materialize, developments centring on the three actor groups can be expected in the future. Although the federal government has withdrawn from the financing of hospital infrastructures and high-tech medical equipment, it has by no means withdrawn entirely from hospital policy-making, as some provisions of the new BPflV indicate.

Set in a broader context, most makers of macro-policy in the hospital field have been flexible and have adapted to changing circumstances. They formed new coalitions when necessary. The new coalitions in support of the Bayern-Vertrag and its imitators in Hesse, Lower Saxony and Berlin, or the anti-hospital lobby, would not have been possible several years ago. The strategic policy actors were willing even to change strategies, if and when new political and economic constellations required them to do so. In the hospital area elements of innovative behaviour, notably among the medical profession, coexist with considerable institutional and structural inertia in the policy-making system. Inertia is plausibly ascribed to the continued influence of the same set of political forces which historically have played leading roles in policy and implementation, and to distinct regional and local traditions that are very much alive.

To summarize, the institutional and structural limits to policy choices and reforms are likely to remain as significant in the future as they have been in the past. If decisions are made, they are likely to continue the traditional style. Compromises on substance are preferred over institutional reforms, and sectoral and incremental approaches are more likely than radical cures.

Note

I gratefully acknowledge financial support from the Präsidium of the Wissenschafts-zentrum Berlin, its International Institute of Management, and the Institut für Informatik and Systemforschung-Medis in Munich. I also thank Fritz Scharpf, Friedhart Hegner, Meinolf Dierkes, Georg Thurn, Detlef Schwefel and Wilhelm van Eimeren.

8

Physicians' Professional Autonomy
in the Welfare State:
Endangered or Preserved?

Marian Döhler

The Problem: Physicians and the Welfare State Dilemma

Throughout Western welfare states physicians are being confronted with increasing pressure on their professional autonomy. This development is due to a mechanism which could be described as the 'welfare state dilemma'. If the physicians of a country participate in a publicly or at least para-fiscally financed health insurance programme, this will significantly change the conditions of their professional activities. On the one hand the doctors' market capacity will be considerably expanded; on the other hand, physicians will become the object of economically motivated attempts by welfare state agencies to control their behaviour. This has been the case particularly since the maturation of the welfare state has led to a significant resource transfer into the health care system, whereby the clinical working process has lost its purely medical character and become a measure of macro-economic significance. For example, it is estimated that at least 80 percent of the overall health care costs are generated by physicians' medical decisions (Schroeder 1980: 23).

The significance of physicians as cost generators is not simply a problem of doctors' fees, although they are often directly linked with the number of procedures, but is rather a result of the resource allocating function of clinical decisions. The crucial point is that diagnosis and therapy patterns of physicians determine the costs of cures to a large degree. This can be inferred from the 'crisis of the welfare state' which has, in the long run, reduced the ability and the willingness of public and private payers to finance rapidly growing health care costs. Thus it can be expected that cost control efforts, immediately aimed at physicians' medical behaviour, would reach a new degree of intensity.

This assumption is based not only on consideration of economic constraints, but on two additional factors. First, the decline of the formerly high esteem of the medical profession has occurred because the limitations of orthodox medicine became apparent through such problems as iatrogenesis and the generally decreasing marginal utility of public health care investments. These problems have been criticized by such writers as Ivan Illich and Thomas McKeown. The declining trust in modern medicine is significant because it shakes severely one of the most important shields for the superior position of physicians in the health care system – their medical expertise. Therefore, the clinical autonomy of physicians is no longer sacrosanct and could be exposed to the pressure of economic constraints. Secondly, scientific and technological developments in the area of electronic data processing have laid the whole medical working process bare. This capacity also increases the possibility of standardizing medical procedures in their economic aspects.

Following the dictum of Rudolf Klein that 'the Welfare State is the residual beneficiary of the Growth State' (1980: 29), control procedures which reach to the core of professional autonomy were superfluous as long as the economic growth rates of the post-war period counterbalanced the costs of the medical working process. Owing to the absence of such growth rates, and the presence of concurrently enhanced public involvement in the financing of health services, distributional conflicts are now occurring. Therefore physicians' freedom of medical choice is inevitably becoming a focal point for public cost control activities.

The term 'professional autonomy' refers in this case to the ability of the physician to make autonomous decisions concerning the contents and the conditions of the medical working process (Freidson 1973: 368). This definition takes into account the distinctions between collective power, which mainly refers to the political and economic actions of organized medicine, and the individual powers of doctors, consisting to a large extent of freedom in the medical decision-making process. From this definition it follows that a loss of professional autonomy occurs when the physician is forced to take into account external – especially economic – calculations. Although economic factors were never completely absent from medical decisions (Luft 1983), they have not previously had a dominant influence. This, however, would be the case, and professional autonomy would certainly be endangered, if utilization reviews, systems of economic monitoring, and/or therapy plans, all based on efficiency criteria, were imposed on the physician.

In the struggle for control over medical care, physicians have advanced the argument that expansion of health and welfare

bureaucracies almost automatically causes a restriction of professional autonomy, which in turn leads to a reduction in the quality of
medical services. In most countries, especially in Germany, this has
been a powerful argument against increased control over the
medical profession by public authorities. Interestingly enough, the
assumption that professional autonomy in particular is restricted by
the integration of the physician into the machinery of welfare
bureaucracies is not only a vital part of the credo of the medical
profession itself, but also a commonly held opinion within the social
sciences. This opinion has been based upon evidence from studies of
individual countries, owing to a lack of international comparisons
(Charles 1976; Björck 1977; Baier 1978; Tiemann 1983). The above-
mentioned welfare state dilemma also seems to buttress this opinion.
If this is true, then a distancing of physicians from the welfare state
enhances professional autonomy; conversely, proximity to welfare
state agencies inevitably reduces the scope of professional autonomy. But there are two factors which make the relevance of this
assumption questionable.

First, for some years doctors in the USA have been exposed to a
severe challenge to their professional autonomy. It is even
suggested that clinical autonomy is largely a fading illusion in the
United States (see chapter 9). This fact is at first glance astonishing,
because US physicians were long regarded by medical sociologists,
political scientists, and economists as the best example of an interest
group which was able to achieve its economic and professional goals
(Alford 1975; Goodman 1980b). Furthermore, a restriction of
professional autonomy was usually considered the necessary outcome of state intervention, as in the case of the introduction of
national health insurance. However, one of the most remarkable
features of the US health care system is precisely the lack of
national health insurance and the related welfare state interventions
as they exist in Western Europe. Therefore, the predominantly
private US health care system ought to preserve a high degree of
professional autonomy. Secondly, there are several (mostly critical)
research reports which indicate that the medical profession in
different countries, despite a highly developed welfare state
bureaucracy, has been able to preserve its autonomy in the clinical
working process (Mechanic 1976: 30).

Because of these apparently contradictory facts and opinions, this
chapter challenges the popular assumption that an increased welfare
state, that is a 'socialization' of the health care system, inevitably
causes a loss of professional autonomy. This thesis will be examined
in the light of the following questions:

1   To what extent were physicians able to preserve their profess-

ional autonomy in welfare states with different degrees of organizational density in the health care sector?
2 On which mechanisms is the stabilization or the destabilization of professional autonomy based?
3 Which conditions must be fulfilled to preserve professional autonomy to an extent which does not affect the quality of health care?

As far as possible, only office-based physicians will be considered because the working situation in hospitals usually differs significantly from that in private practice. Of course, this subdivision is feasible only in countries with clear boundaries between the two sectors, as is the case in Germany.

Comparing Physicians' Professional Autonomy in Five Welfare States

The countries which are considered here are the USA, the Federal Republic of Germany, the UK, France, and Sweden. This choice is based on the health care system typology of Mark Field (1980). In accordance with this typology, welfare states with a low (USA), a medium (Germany, France), and a high (UK, Sweden) degree of organizational density in the health care sector have been chosen. The differentiation between different degrees of organizational density is based on the level of market dominance or state dominance in the health care system. Therefore, three ideal types could be identified: a mainly market-based model with no comprehensive public health insurance; a restricted market model in which, owing to the existence of a national health insurance, that is a monopolistic payment structure, only the sector of health care providers has retained some market mechanisms; and a state-dominated model in which both sectors are a state responsibility.

It can be expected that the following factors are responsible to some extent for determining the degree of professional autonomy: (1) the organizational structure of the health care system, (2) the dominant health policy and welfare state ideologies, (3) the power position and structure of the major medical associations, and (4) existing procedures for negotiating doctors' remuneration, and supervision or monitoring systems for clinical decision-making. Each country will therefore be analysed under these criteria.

United States: physicians and the free market
The US health care system is the only one which can still be defined as pluralistic in Field's typology. In the US there is no national health insurance scheme which covers the vast majority of the

population as there is in most Western European welfare states. Rather, the US health care system is predominantly private and highly decentralized. Although the federal government finances a significant part of the health services, control over these public funds is left extensively to the private sector.

In this health care system, the medical profession held a very influential position which was unique in the Western world for a long time. For example, under the pressure of the physicians' well-organized and powerful lobby, the American Medical Association (AMA), several attempts to introduce a national health insurance were thwarted because this would have unavoidably led to greater public control (Starr 1982). Moreover, on the basis of the lobbying capacities of organized medicine, the health insurance programmes of Medicare (for the old) and Medicaid (for the poor), introduced in 1965, were not connected with an intensified public authority to control physicians' behaviour. To obtain the agreement of the AMA for the passing of the Medicare/Medicaid bill, legislators were forced to concede to the medical profession permission to charge fees under the provision that they would be 'usual, customary, and reasonable' (Marmor 1973: 80). The AMA was also successful in endorsing the 'prohibition against any interference clause' (Björkman, this volume), which only allows a very weak monitoring of physicians' behaviour. Because, moreover, both programmes are administered through fiscal intermediaries, consisting of private health insurance carriers, the government's ability to control the costs of these programmes is even less.

The fact that Medicare and Medicaid were mostly responsible for a rapid cost explosion in the health care sector (which put increasing strains on the federal and the state budgets), however, led to the passage of a bill in 1972 which was designed to build up so-called professional standards review organizations (PSROs). In order to ensure a high quality of care, these regulatory agencies were designed to monitor physicians' prescriptions for Medicare and Medicaid patients. At the same time, they were to function as a check on cost control. However, because the AMA was able to influence the legislative process, the administration of the PSROs was left entirely to regional medical societies (Starr 1982: 400). Therefore, the PSROs were hardly ready to perform this function. Similar judgements could be made about subsequent regulatory laws, such as the Health Planning Act of 1974 (Starr 1982: 401).

It could be argued that, until the 1970s, the political power of US physicians was mainly based on their potential ability to refuse to participate in public health programmes and, additionally, on deeply rooted public and congressional wariness of state intervention in general. The veto-like power of the AMA corresponds to the fact that public health care agencies in the US have few instruments to influence or even to monitor physicians' behaviour. In other words, state interventions up to now have not entailed a restriction of physicians' professional autonomy, mainly because they could be either neutralized or completely rejected by the AMA.

Strangely enough, the inability of the federal government to control health care costs ultimately led to three developments which constitute a serious challenge to physicians' professional autonomy. First, since the mid 1970s private business firms have developed an intensified interest in holding down the cost explosion. This involvement is based on the fact that some employers in the US pay up to 90 percent of the health insurance premiums of their employees. Logically, private firms are trying to curb health care costs in a more radical way than public bureaucracies ever could. Business interests are therefore watching the clinical working process of physicians in various ways. They are trying to negotiate the use of cheaper methods of diagnosis and therapy with health care providers, that is physicians and hospitals. Private peer review firms are appointed to control and if necessary to 'adjust' the practices of physicians. Business coalitions, that is voluntary associations of business enterprises, educate their members to deal with reluctant physicians and hospitals (Döhler 1985).

Secondly, the rapid cost explosion has transformed the health care sector from a cottage industry into an attractive object for commercial investors (Starr 1982; Wohl 1984). Because of the low welfare state density in the US and the ingrained preference of the incumbent conservative health policy-makers for commercial health care providers and insurers, there is little resistance to the economization of good health. Thus over the past few years a profit-oriented medical-industrial complex has been evolving which consists mainly of large-scale hospital and HMO chains (Wohl 1984). The numerous advantages in marketing and economics of scale that this complex has over the non-profit sector accelerates the rapid expansion of commercial health care facilities. At the same time, in part due to receding opportunities for practising solo and the growing oversupply of medical graduates, physicians are increasingly forced into financial dependence upon the medical-industrial complex (Derber 1984). Because profit, in other words the cheap 'production' of health, is the driving force in commercial health care facilities, physicians are exposed to intensive monitoring of their diagnosis and therapy patterns by sophisticated computer information systems and utilization reviews (Fuchs 1982). These practices might result in a loss of professional autonomy if, for example, physicians are forced to comply with fixed therapy plans, or if deviations, even for prescribing too little, are penalized (Starr 1982: 420–49).

Thus, physicians' victories of the past shaped the defeats of the present: 'The great irony is that opposition of the doctors and hospitals to public control of public programs set in motion entrepreneurial forces that may end up depriving both private doctors and local voluntary hospitals of their traditional autonomy' (Starr 1982: 445). Success in preventing close control of their professional autonomy by public authorities brings US doctors increasingly under the much more vigorous control of private enterprise.

Thirdly, under pressure from the accelerating cost spiral the federal government introduced so-called diagnostic-related groups (DRGs), which were designed to be a prospective payment mechanism (as opposed to the former retrospective system) for hospital services which are paid by the Medicare programme. After an unusually short period of congressional discussions, the DRG scheme was enacted in 1982 as an amendment to the Medicare bill. Contrary to the former retrospective payment mechanism, DRGs categorize all clinical procedures into 467 diagnostic groups with a fixed price for each. In the US this is widely interpreted as a revolution in health service payment because the state determines, by price setting, the remuneration of each medical therapy and thereby forces hospital administrators to enter the medical decision-making process (Dunham and Marone 1984). On the political and ideological level the process of subordinating the medical profession to economic constraints is supported by the currently prevailing market reform advocates in the Reagan administration and in Congress. As opposed to traditional conservatives, market reformers are not concerned with the autonomy of physicians. Therefore, the erosion of professional autonomy in the US will continue in the foreseeable future.

Germany: the advantages of health policy corporatism
The German health care system, as opposed to the American, is mainly based on a statutory health insurance (GKV) which covers the vast majority of the population. The German GKV is the prototype of a social insurance system; it consists of nearly 1,300 sickness funds, which have the status of bodies of public law, and which are financed in equal parts by the premiums from employers and employees (Stone 1980). The dominant ideology is so-called self-administration, which means that the sickness funds are

administered by equal numbers of elected officials from the associations of employers and employees. The self-administration ideology also holds for physicians' organizations. This system is due to a very complex legal code, the *Reichsversicherungsordnung* (RVO), which regulates in detail the functions and competencies of the different actors in the German health care system.

As a result of the self-administration ideology, physicians in Germany are represented by a three-tiered organizational system which is vested with extensive self-governing rights for the medical profession (Rauskolb 1976). Physicians' chambers (*Ärztekammern*), of which membership is compulsory, mostly deal with matters such as professional ethics, the continuation of medical education, and professional tribunals. The various private medical associations are mainly organs to represent and to articulate physicians' political interests. Far and away the most important of these organizations in this context are the eighteen regional associations of insurance doctors (*Kassenärztliche Vereinigung*: KV). Each physician who wants to participate in the GKV is required to be a member of one of these public law institutions, which are administered solely by physicians.

Among the functions of the KV is the negotiation of physicians' reimbursement with the regional associations of sickness funds and the administration of the aggregate reimbursement (*Gesamtvergütung*) (Schülke 1977) which, as a result of the annual negotiations, is transferred from the sickness funds and used to pay the member doctors according to the services they have rendered to the insured patients (Glaser 1978: 98; Stone 1980: 95). According to the rules of the RVO, each KV has to consider the principle of economic efficiency. In particular this means that the KV is responsible for the efficiency of the prescription patterns of its members, the physicians. Therefore, each KV has a review board which monitors the economic soundness of physicians' prescribing behaviour (Stone 1980: 105). Although there is a range of different sanctions against physicians with excessive prescriptions – for example cutback of reimbursement – until 1977 the review boards had no leverage to intervene in questions of professional autonomy. First, the monitoring process was the sole responsibility of physicians. Officials of the sickness funds were also represented on the boards, but only as consulting members. Secondly, the criterion for charging an individual physician with overprescribing is that the claims exceed the statistical average by more than 40 percent. These procedures have enabled physicians only marginally to take economic calculations into account (Stone 1980: 116).

Nevertheless, recent legislation, especially the Health Care Cost

Containment Act (KVKG) of 1977, has been interpreted by several authors as a severe threat to the clinical freedom of physicians (Baier 1978: 115; Hamm 1980; Nord 1982: 63), because a universal expenditure ceiling is imposed on physicians' reimbursement which apparently forces doctors to take economic measures into account and, additionally, because the governing procedures of the review boards were modified.

With the KVKG a corporatist negotiating institution, the Konzertierte Aktion im Gesundheitswesen (KAG), was introduced (Wiesenthal 1981), which might in theory have threatened the professional autonomy of physicians. The major function of the KAG, in which the associations of physicians, hospitals (since 1982), sickness funds, and the different levels of government are represented on a voluntary basis, is to recommend an annual increase of health care expenditures, including physicians' reimbursement, which is linked to the annual average increase of wages and salaries (*Grundlohnsumme*). The sickness funds and KVs are expected to negotiate fee increases to fit these recommendations. Although this subordination of the health care costs to measures of economic development represents a striking turning point in German health care policy, it need not be viewed as an assault on professional autonomy because the KAG has the capacity only to recommend, not to enforce, a certain level of health care expenditures. If the recommendation is exceeded, no sanctions against physicians are possible. Consequently, in order to strengthen the cost containment capacity of the sickness funds, the KVKG required that the funds must be henceforth equally represented in the review boards. The law also required an annual change of each board's chairman, who has the deciding vote in case of ties. However, recent research on the actual impact of the efficiency review indicates that even this change in the power structure of economic monitoring has had no significant affect on physicians' behaviour (Döhler 1986). This is attributable to the complex guidelines for penalizing a physician for inefficiency, as well as to the dominating role which officials of the KV still play in the review procedure. Accordingly, sanctions are difficult for the review boards to handle, even under the increased influence of cost-conscious sickness funds.

Thus, the autonomy of German physicians remains unchallenged, to a significant degree, thanks to the twofold organizational integration of physicians into the welfare state network. On the macroeconomic level, their participation in a corporatist negotiating institution serves as a buffer against possible threats to professional autonomy through the negotiating mechanism of the KAG; this facilitates package deals between government and physicians, such as moderate fee increases in return for restricted access to medical schools. On the regional and local level the extensive self-governing authority, which is legally as well as structurally established in the KV, makes changes in the power structure extremely difficult to implement. Interventions by the federal government, which might otherwise impair physicians' clinical freedom, have to be implemented within the existing structures. Such is the case with the above-mentioned monitoring of prescription patterns, which are very much in favour of the physicians' economic and professional needs.

United Kingdom: physicians and socialized medicine
Since the turn of the century, the medical profession in Western countries has successfully twisted the term 'socialized medicine' to prevent policy developments which might lead to greater public authority in the health care system. From this point of view the introduction of the British National Health Service (NHS) in 1948 was a unique achievement among capitalist nations. Until Italy launched its Servizio Sanitario Nazionale in 1980, the NHS formed the only health care system among Western nations which was based on a centrally determined and administered budget, almost completely financed by general taxation, and intended to provide free provision of medical services to the entire population (Klein 1983a). This function is carried out by a complicated and hierarchically ordered administrative structure which is part of the central government. Market forces and even the insurance principle, sometimes viewed as the organizational basis of the modern welfare state, are completely excluded from health care, with the exception of a small but increasingly important private sector.

However, even if the term 'socialized medicine' might be an appropriate characterization of the NHS, some major qualifications should be emphasized. First, on the level of ideology, the NHS is not simply a socialist victory, but more the outcome of a 'radically managerial ideology' (Klein 1983a: 25) arising from the intellectual consensus of the two major political parties. Secondly, the British health care system was not entirely socialized by the introduction of the NHS. This was only the case with hospitals; physicians were dealt with in a different way.

Today there are two major groups of practising physicians within the NHS. General practitioners serve as gatekeepers to the NHS (Klein 1983a: 87) because they are usually the first point of contact between the patient and the medical system. If specialist services and access to sophisticated medical technology are needed, the general practitioner refers the patient to a specialist. These so-called consultants, who are exclusively located in a hospital setting, represent the second group of physicians. As of the mid 1960s, when the first major payment dispute occurred (Marmor and Thomas 1972: 428), all British physicians are economically represented by the union-like British Medical Association (BMA).

Only the general practitioners are employed on a salaried basis by the NHS. Consultants have the option to work as part-time or full-time employees of the NHS with a fixed salary. The hospital doctor's income, however, is not entirely dependent on the fixed NHS budget. This is the consequence of one of the most important and still disputed concessions made to secure the agreement of the medical profession for the introduction of the NHS: the right of hospital doctors to maintain highly profitable private beds in public hospitals for the use of privately insured or fee-for-service patients (Klein 1983a: 118). As opposed to consultants, the general practitioners are not employed directly by the NHS but work on a contract basis. Depending on the panel list of their patients, usually about 2,200, they receive a capitation payment from the Family Practitioner Committee, the administrative tier of the NHS which is responsible for securing ambulatory care.

Since the introduction of the NHS, arrangements and amounts of remuneration for physicians have been negotiated directly by the participants. This period of negotiations between the central government, represented by the Department of Health and Social Security (DHSS), the BMA and the Royal College of Surgeons was terminated in 1962. From that point on, annual increases in salaries and capitation payments have been determined by the Review Body for Doctors' and Dentists' Remuneration. This is an independent but state-financed agency which consists of a chairman and six 'eminent persons of experience in various fields of national life' (Glaser 1978: 164), who are appointed by the cabinet, usually with the approval of the BMA, and are supported by a civil service staff from the Cabinet Office. The Review Body stands in the tradition of the so-called quangos (quasi non-governmental organizations). Therefore the agency is independent of governmental orders, but on the other hand its decision-making power does not include the right to fix physicians' remuneration. The function of the Review Body is solely 'to advise the Prime Minister on the remuneration of doctors and dentists taking any part in the National Health Service' (Levitt 1977: 105). Only if the recommendations are accepted by the cabinet can they come into force.

The Review Body determines doctors' remuneration by weighing the demands of physicians' associations (mainly the BMA), the proposals of the DHSS, current budget plans, and the evaluation of statistical material such as changes in the cost of living or expenses in general practices (Levitt 1977: 105; Glaser 1978: 169). Although the intention is that these recommendations represent a kind of common denominator of physicians and the government, it is clear that the calculations of the Review Body have to take into account economic measures which are inextricably entangled with the budgetary constraints of the NHS. Under this system, the feasibility of a physician-induced cost explosion is to a large extent eliminated, chiefly by the methods of remuneration – that is salary and capitation, which create no financial incentives for the doctor to prescribe more than necessary – and the determination of that remuneration by an independent agency, which is inevitably forced to consider the fixed budget of the NHS. The latter serves especially as a mechanism to channel the sometimes aggressively demanded income increases into the realms of the economically feasible.

Therefore, it seems to be a logical development that British physicians still enjoy a very high degree of clinical autonomy (Elston 1977; Tolliday 1978). Although this autonomy has aroused vehement criticism for disregarding consumer needs (Robson 1973) or for being inefficient (Maynard 1984), it is among the most sacrosanct ideologies in British health politics. Review agencies or controlling bodies for overseeing the prescribing patterns of physicians are largely unknown in Britain. This is attributable to the fact that 'because the NHS has a strict system of financial control over the total amount of resources allocated, it has so far not had to devise a system of trying to control individual medical decisions' (Klein 1977: 172). Interestingly enough, the only prescribing reviews – constituting, however, no real threat to physicians' autonomy – are imposed on the general practitioners, which is the group of physicians in the NHS least integrated into the bureaucratic structure of the British welfare state (Ham 1985: 53).

France: la médecine libérale and national health insurance
As is the case with Germany, in the French health care system the financing structures are a public responsibility, whereas medical care is provided mainly by private physicians and by a mix of public and private hospitals. Approximately 99 percent of the French population is covered by a compulsory health insurance scheme consisting of three national sickness funds, of which the Caisse Nationale d'Assurance Maladie des Travailleurs Salariés (CNAM), insuring about 75 percent of the population, is the most important (Rodwin 1981: 19). The different *caisses* are financed by the contributions of employers and employees and are also jointly

administered. This centralized arrangement has been in effect since the social security reform of 1967 succeeded a highly decentralized and complex mixture of local sickness funds.

The reform of 1967 has not only strengthened the centralized control of the government over the health care system, by subordinating the sickness funds under the direct supervision of the Ministries of Health and Finance, but has also brought about a significant change in the administration of the funds. The labour-dominated boards were replaced and labour unions and employers became equally represented (Rodwin 1982: 301). The 1967 reform brought about changes that affected physicians as well. Instead of regional health insurance carriers, from whom they had won significant concessions in previous years, they now had to face the CNAM, a powerful bargaining agency with an increased interest in cost containment as a result of close ministerial supervision.

The current shape of the French health care system is the result of a historical struggle between those interests which are represented by the two conflicting ideologies of liberalism and solidarity (Rodwin 1981: 18). Since the French state abandoned its *laissez-faire* attitudes towards health policy after World War II (Rodwin 1982), liberalism is now only present in the concept of *la médecine libérale*. This term refers to a set of rules which physicians regard as indispensable for sufficient medical care: 'the patient's free choice of doctor, the physician's freedom of prescription, professional confidentiality, and the fee-for-service payment' (Godt 1985: 158). The concept of *solidarité*, on the other hand, was one of the most influential values leading to the introduction of a national health insurance in 1945. The responsibility of the state to ensure access to a sufficient level of medical care for the whole population and *la médecine libérale* served as the basis for most health policy conflicts (Sandier and Stephan 1983: 67).

One of the most striking examples is the involvement of the government in the area of regulating physicians' fees. This began with the May 1960 decree, as a result of which the medical profession was forced for the first time to accept departmental negotiations (*conventions*), subject to government consent, between the medical union, the Confédération des Syndicats Médicaux Français (CSMF), and regional social security authorities over fee schedules (Steudler 1977: 190). The *convention* lays down in detail the relations between physicians and sickness funds, and also contains the *nomenclature*, an annually renewed fee schedule (Glaser 1978: 40). The crucial innovation in the 1960 decree was that if no collective agreements could be reached, physicians would be allowed to contract on an individual basis with the CNAM.

Because this rendered the CSMF superfluous as a bargaining agent, and because physicians until that time were free to set fees, serious internal conflict arose within the medical profession on the issue of accepting the *conventions*.

Although the *conventions* contained a ceiling for fees, and thereby deviated from the sacred principles of *la médecine libérale*, most physicians accepted them. Those physicians who rejected the system of regional *conventions*, for the most part affluent urban specialists, formed the insurgent Fédération des Médecins de France (FMF). In turn, the ensuing rivalry between the FMF and the CSMF created a dilemma for the medical profession because the government played the two medical unions against each other. In the 1971 negotiations about a new *convention*, the CSMF regained the function of speaking for physicians *vis-à-vis* the CNAM. Nevertheless, the medical profession was seriously weakened by the internal cleavage between the two rival associations. The CSMF achieved significant success by acquiring 'a solemn commitment of the government' (Godt 1985: 158) to respect the concept of *la médecine libérale* in the 1971 *convention*, but in the 1976 negotiations the FMF signed the agreement alone, thereby forcing the CSMF to follow suit. The same happened in the 1980 negotiations (Godt 1985: 162).

But it was not only the division between the two medical unions that reduced the bargaining power of the medical profession. Because the *convention* of 1971 was negotiated as a national agreement which applied to all office-based physicians, the ability of the medical unions to avoid national agreement on physicians' fee increases was halted. Cost control efforts had become a matter of concern with macro-economic significance. This had been especially brought into focus by the oil crisis of 1973, which marked the end of post-war economic prosperity and forced the central government to implement a tighter cost containment policy. Owing to this development, as well as to the above-mentioned cleavage between the two medical unions, in 1977 physicians were not able to negotiate fee increases above the inflation rate and their income in real terms declined for the first time (Godt 1985: 160). Facing an ever-growing budget deficit the CNAM, since 1978, has been trying to keep the fee increases below the inflation rate. More recently, after the 1981 Socialist election victory, a fee schedule was introduced in the 1981 *convention*, which was closely linked to government-fixed economic measures. This cost containment policy proved successful enough to balance the 1983 budget (Godt 1985: 166) and relieved physicians from state intervention which might have impaired their freedom in clinical decisions. Although a reduction in professional autonomy remains a possibility (Rodwin 1981: 38; Herzlich 1982: 252), French physicians hitherto have preserved theirs.

The French case suggests that the relative success of governmental cost containment has played an important part in protecting physicians from the intensified economic monitoring which could have been a result of the 1971 *convention*. Since then, individual medical profiles of each participating physician have been obtainable from the data pools of the sickness funds. The original aim of the profiles was to generate self-discipline within the medical profession by exposing the physician himself to data about his excessive prescriptions (Rodwin 1982: 301). Although this was largely a symbolic enterprise, a technical tool for restricting the therapeutic freedom of physicians had been irretrievably created (Herzlich 1982: 251; Rodwin 1981: 31). Therefore, in France, the intervention of a strong welfare state into the health policy field (Steudler 1984) has diluted the physicians' bargaining power in order to achieve moderate increases in fees, and has thereby reduced the need for cost containment measures that might result in a loss in professional autonomy (Herzlich 1982: 250).

Sweden: towards a salaried profession

The ideological and organizational principles of the Swedish health care system largely form a model which is close to the ideal national health service. Although there are still some elements of their preceding health insurance model, as of the mid 1970s the health care system had been transformed by a 'silent socialization' into a quasi-public health service (Glaser 1978: 134). This could be verified in three ways. First, the main ideological orientation of Swedish health policy is based for the most part on the government's commitment to secure equality of access to the full range of medical care for the entire population. Therefore, all Swedish citizens are covered by a compulsory health insurance consisting of 23 regional sickness funds.

Secondly, the Swedish medical profession has become corporatized, since the vast majority of physicians work in the organizational context of overwhelmingly public-owned hospitals. The number of private practices is declining steadily. Today fewer than 7 percent of practitioners are not employed by the state, and less than 5 percent of the hospitals are privately owned (Hammerström and Janlert 1983: 244). As a result of the great importance which the hospital has in Swedish medicine, only a small percentage of practices are office-based district physicians providing primary non-specialist care.

Thirdly, by far the most important agencies for the health care system are the 23 regional county councils (*landsting*) which are responsible for planning, financing, and supplying hospital as well as primary medical care in their area (Hessler and Twaddle 1982). The sickness funds, which evolved from the private health insurance carriers during the 1950s, are public agencies which merely retain the function of collecting the contributions from employers and employees and allocating these funds for the payment of medical services. They are under the close supervision of the national government and have no significant decision-making rights of their own (Glaser 1978: 137). This means that no para-fiscal, quasi-public or even private institution but rather a regional branch of the state is responsible for the supply and allocation of health services. Therefore the counties run most hospitals and health centres, and employ the district physicians. These services are financed by the contributions collected by the sickness funds, by taxes levied by the counties, and by additional grants from the national government (Carder and Klingeberg 1980: 146).

In accordance with the Swedish health care system, and the predominantly salaried status of physicians, the medical profession is organized in the union-like Swedish Medical Association (SLF), which has about 90 percent of all physicians as members. As a result, the SLF has a representation monopoly for negotiations over salaries and working conditions with public employers (Glaser 1978: 139). Within the SMA the association of junior doctors (SYLF), attributable to their growing number, has become the most important group. Although the SYLF as an autonomous organiz-ation has no bargaining functions, and all their members are simultaneously in the SLF, it has exerted great influence on the health policy attitudes of the SMA. Since the mid 1950s the SYLF members have attained a significantly stronger position on the SLF's executive committee (Heidenheimer 1980: 126). The SYLF leaders contributed considerably to the transformation of the SLF from a professional association into a trade union with 'lesser concern with protecting professional "autonomy" or the status distinctions between medicine and other occupational groups, and greater con-cern with successful economic bargaining results' (Heidenheimer 1980: 135).

It is necessary to mention the SYLF dominance within the SLF to understand the modes of policy-making surrounding the so-called seven crowns reform (SCR) of 1970, the most important post-war legislative action concerning the situation of Swedish physicians. The outcome of the SCR was that government-employed physicians, that is 90 percent of all physicians, were totally excluded from financial transactions with the patient. Prior to 1970, physicians had been allowed to practise part-time on a fee-for-service basis. The patient had to pay the physician directly and was then reimbursed at a rate of 75 percent of the fee schedule by the sickness funds. Henceforth, the fee-for-service principle was eliminated by putting government-employed physicians on a full salary and prohibiting at the same time the charging of additional fees. Instead, the patient had to pay a fixed fee of seven crowns for each out-patient visit, a figure which has since been increased considerably. Furthermore, the income differences between the various groups of physicians, which had caused internal conflicts within the SLF during the 1960s, were reduced. Almost needless to say, the SCR was the reaction to the unsuccessful efforts to control the health care cost explosion by means of fee schedules (Shenkin 1973: 557).

Although this radical change in physicians' remuneration was somewhat disputed within the medical profession, especially because of income reductions for some specialists with above-average incomes and the abolition of the fee-for-service principle, the SLF finally accepted the SCR. The agreement of the medical profession to be almost entirely socialized is only understandable if one imagines the slow transformation of the SMA towards a professional trade union with corresponding collectivist attitudes. This had led to a situation in which, 'from the perspective of the SLF leadership [under the influence of the SYLF], the SCR provided an opportunity to solidify and institutionalize the new role' (Carder and Klingeberg 1980: 169) as a trade union.

Even though it is assumed that, at least since the SCR, Swedish physicians have been under total government control (Björck 1977), their professional autonomy has been left untouched (Hessler and Twaddle 1986: 139; Saltman 1983). Of course, the ability of physicians to determine their income was strongly reduced by the elimination of the fee-for-service principle. But, on the other hand, while the government received a great opportunity to control physicians' income via negotiations over salaries with the SLF, other forms of health care cost controls, possibly challenging physicians' autonomy, have been abandoned. The only incursion into professional autonomy worth mentioning has been the setting up of a Health and Medical Services Disciplinary Board, a central government agency which inquires into patient complaints levelled against doctors in order to ensure quality of care (Lane and Arvidson, this volume). But even if physicians anticipate possible sanctions in their day-to-day work, it is unlikely that the controls of the Board significantly reduce their clinical latitude. This is because controls are mainly aimed at rare malpractice cases – which would be investigated even if the Board did not exist – and because 'professional dominance' still shapes the doctor–patient relationship in Sweden (Hessler and Twaddle 1986: 139).

Discussion

There can be no doubt that economic decision-making rights, as well as the ability to define the direction of health policy, significantly shifted away from the medical profession as the welfare state expanded, and there is still the impending danger of extra-professional control of physicians' clinical behaviour. However at present, with the remarkable exception of the US, physicians in the countries under review have been able to preserve their professional autonomy to a large extent. This leads to the conclusion that, as opposed to the commonly held opinion, there is no positive correlation between the degree of welfare state development and a reduced professional autonomy of physicians. This assumption gives rise to the question of which factors are responsible for the stabilization or destabilization of professional autonomy in the countries reviewed.

Prior to answering this question, it is necessary to make reference to the limitations of the research findings at hand. First of all physicians themselves, and also most economists, tend to define professional autonomy mainly as economic freedom. However, this chapter is based on a more restricted definition. Only the conditions of the medical working process, chiefly the freedom of clinical decisions, were taken into account. Therefore conclusions drawn here are only valid if this narrower definition is accepted. Secondly, a restriction of physicians' autonomy could also be caused by factors other than welfare state intervention. To mention only the most important: an integration of physicians into larger medical facilities, like hospitals or health centres, might be connected with increased control of clinical behaviour either by peer review or by administratively imposed controls. Furthermore, physicians' decision-making rights might be restricted by the penetration of para-professionals into the area of medical care or increased consumer participation (Haug and Lavin 1983). Finally, physicians' rights to decide autonomously over patients' treatment might be impaired by court decisions, as in the US where the number of malpractice suits is increasing astronomically, or by the growing number of laws curtailing doctors' leeway (Müller 1979). If professional autonomy is restricted in a country, factors like those mentioned above have to be distinguished from those of welfare state expansion.

On reconsidering the previous sections, it becomes clear that in each of the five countries different arrangements have developed in the attempt to balance the conflicting requirements of physicians' professional autonomy and increasingly drained health budgets. Two features are mainly responsible for the conditions stabilizing professional autonomy. In the most socialized health care systems of the UK and Sweden, the income of physicians was largely separated from the medical working process by introducing capitation payments or salaries, whereas in France and Germany the strain placed by physicians on the available health care budgets is lightened by negotiations over fees. The medical profession in Germany is resistant to incursions into its autonomy because of its extensive self-government rights, as well as by means of corporatist decision-making for national health policy developments. On the other hand, in France the politicization of health policy has led to state intervention, mainly aimed at physicians' payments, causing a dispersion of the professions' corporate power which in turn has enabled the central government to impose remarkable cost containment measures on physicians.

The question remains of what, if anything, these countries have in common concerning the mechanisms of preserving physicians' professional autonomy despite economic constraints. First, in all cases, governmental regulations of physicians' income serve as a cost containment instrument which substitutes for restrictions on the freedom of medical decision-making, even if there is only a marginal impact on cost containment. It looks as if existing cost containment institutions and procedures, in particular regulations of doctors' income, lead away from incursions into professional autonomy. Organized negotiations are lacking in the US, whereas physicians in Germany, France, the UK and Sweden are linked partly to economic constraints by collective bargaining. Accordingly, a reduction of professional autonomy could be avoided best if physicians were able to restrain or at least postpone their economic demands. Or to exaggerate the argument: professional autonomy is preserved best where physicians' financial freedom is restricted most. However, this overstated formulation should be understood as a tendency and not as a hard fact.

Second, doctor–state relations are institutionalized in different ways: either by means of organizational arrangements, as is the case of the KAG in Germany and the Review Body in the UK, or by regular negotiations between public authorities and the medical profession, as can be observed in Sweden and France. Owing to the fact that physicians themselves are obviously unable to behave efficiently, either public or private institutional structures and regulations are required to facilitate income increases not exceeding a crucial point. Because the institutionalization of doctor–state relations tends to consist mainly of bargaining over physicians' income, the pressure on professional autonomy is eased. The mere existence of such an institutional network, however, is no indication of the real efficiency of those instruments of cost containment. For example, in Germany the cost explosion has not been halted by means of the KAG, but the participation of physicians in a national effort for cost containment was symbolically effective. By this means, the public became aware that physicians recognized the cost explosion and were willing to share the burden by accepting a ceiling on their incomes. This is a convincing argument against those who advocate reducing physicians' autonomy in order to reduce overall health care expenditures.

One main thesis suggests itself from the previous findings. The expansion of the welfare state in the health care sector, especially under the current conditions of economic scarcity, has reduced physicians' economic power. On the other hand, the simultaneous institutionalization of the doctor–state relationship has served as a protective cover to physicians' professional autonomy, mainly because it has left a sizeable repertoire of strategies for physicians to avoid direct incursions into their autonomy, that is bargaining and self-government. Exactly these mechanisms would be lacking if market forces took control, and thereby efficiency criteria could be directly imposed on physicians, as is the case in the US. Finally, it must be mentioned that scarce resources have resulted in discussions about a reduction of physicians' autonomy in most Western countries, and the tools for closer control are already in existence. Whether these instruments are applied against professional autonomy, of course, depends on future trends in health costs, but also on physicians' willingness to subordinate their income demands to economic constraints. It seems as if physicians in more developed welfare states are better equipped to meet this challenge.

9
Clinical Autonomy in the United Kingdom and the United States: Contrasts and Convergence

Stephen Harrison and Rockwell I. Schulz

The notion of clinical autonomy (or clinical freedom) is at the heart of social scientists' discussions of the medical profession. Sociologists such as Millerson (1964) have seen autonomy as one of the defining traits of the profession. More critical writers such as Freidson (1970) and Johnson (1972), while rejecting the necessity to see professions as they see themselves, have regarded their claims to autonomy as a major component of their ability to dominate non-professionals. Clinical autonomy also figures prominently in the parlance of physicians themselves, especially in reference to contemporary attempts to secure greater managerial control over health services (Levy and Hesse 1985). After all, if professionalism entails autonomy, management (to put it crudely) entails curtailing people's autonomy and controlling them. This remains the case even where methods of control are more subtle than close supervision, perhaps involving the manipulation of corporate cultures (Peters and Waterman 1983).

Yet clinical autonomy remains a subject which has seldom undergone systematic analysis. There can be no systems of absolute clinical autonomy for physicians, since such licence for one physician would entail the right to interfere with another physician's freedom. The significant questions therefore concern: freedom from whom, and to do what? These questions are addressed through recent British and American experiences after clarifying the notion of clinical freedom and briefly tracing the logic by which it has currently become an issue. This chapter analyses the nature of clinical autonomy in Britain and the United States by identifying contrasts which have emerged as a result of their different approaches to three matters: the funding of health services; the remuneration of physicians; and litigation against doctors. A final section examines recent trends in the two countries, which suggest that common perceptions of the need to provide health care more economically are leading to a convergence of their characteristic approaches to clinical autonomy,

The Concept of Clinical Autonomy

In one of the few attempts to undertake empirical research into clinical autonomy, Harrison et al. (1984) found that few of their clinician respondents were able to articulate a coherent definition of the concept. However, Tolliday (1978) has drawn attention to four kinds of claims to autonomy which have been articulated by physicians. These are: the right to independent practice; the right to refuse an individual patient; the responsibility to lead and co-ordinate other health professions; and the overarching primacy of medical knowledge.

The various elements of Tolliday's definition relate the claims of physicians to a series of other actors in the health care arena. These other actors are those characterized by Alford (1975) as the main structural interests in the field of health care politics; for the moment these can be labelled as professionals, consumers and third parties such as governments, managers and payers. Thus, Tolliday's first element refers to relationships between professionals and third parties, her second element to relationships between consumers and professionals, and her other elements to interprofessional relationships.

In the idealized nineteenth-century liberal concept of medicine and commerce, there are no third parties; there is only the direct relationship between the patient and his or her independent family practitioner. In such circumstances, clinical autonomy is not held to be an issue, since both parties have freedom of choice over whether to continue the relationship. If the relationship does continue, it is governed by the long-standing provision of both English (Speller 1965) and American law (Miller 1983) that patients' consent to treatment is required. Ostensibly, therefore, the doctor has no freedom to decide how to treat the patient, although the technological complexity of medicine and the allegedly mystifying tendencies of professionalism (Illich 1977) call into question the patients' ability to give informed consent.

This idealized picture was never wholly accurate since there were always some third parties in the form of hospital owners, friendly societies and the like; but it clearly differed from present-day reality. Although their nature varies from country to country, third parties are now entrenched actors in every health care system in the world. These third parties include payers (insurance companies, provident associations, sickness funds, employers and governments), providers of facilities (hospital owners, governments and charities), their agents and managers, and governments as regulators. It is the increasing importance of these third parties which makes clinical autonomy into an issue, for it raises questions about the extent to which professionals are (or should be) free from control by them. Although intraprofessional relationships are not unproblematic, these have been amply documented elsewhere (Larkin 1983). This chapter therefore concentrates upon professional/third-party relationships.

Paradoxically, the reason that this aspect of clinical autonomy is an issue is that another relationship, that between third parties and consumers, is highly ambiguous. On the one hand, the consumer is concerned to limit the costs of health, since he or she is the ultimate payer for them, whether directly or, more usually, indirectly through taxation, insurance premiums, or sickness fund contributions. On the other hand, the consumer is also concerned to obtain unlimited health care consumption for himself or herself. In practice, where consumers are not wholly or mainly meeting health care cost by out-of-pocket payments, this ambiguity is resolved through the phenomenon of moral hazard (Cairns and Snell 1978), whereby there is little incentive for individual consumers to restrict personal consumption of health care which is financed from a pool of contributions. But if there is no incentive for one consumer to restrict consumption, there is no incentive for any consumer, and therefore the rate of contributions to the pool of finance will tend to rise. Third parties try to restrict this rate of increase in expenditure either because they themselves contribute to it (for example, employers, and governments as financiers of health care), and/or because they consider such increases to be undesirable on other grounds. For example governments, as makers of macro-economic policy, may be concerned with the proportion of domestic product accounted for by health care expenditure.

In Alford's analysis, the professional monopolizers are regarded as the dominant interest because they have been able to defeat the attempts of third parties to control them. But these third parties (the corporate rationalizers in Alford's terms) are the challenging interest, and the relationships between these two sets of actors are likely to be dynamic. By contrast the consumer interest is repressed and inactive.

Clinical Autonomy in the United Kingdom

The private health care sector in Britain is relatively small, amounting to some 2 percent of the total budget (Royal Commission 1979) and being involved mainly in the provision of nursing homes for the elderly, elective surgery, and abortions. In addition, the services of alternative practitioners such as osteopaths and chiropractors are not provided by the National Health Service (NHS). This relatively small private sector provides few employment opportunities, and indeed the majority of private medical care is provided on a part-time basis by physicians already employed by the NHS.

Funding of health services within the public sector is largely from government sources (mainly general taxation), with only some 3 percent raised from charges to the public (Office of Health Economics 1981). Some 65 percent of expenditure is upon hospital services and a further 14 percent on administration and services aimed at supporting patients in their own homes, such as community nursing, midwifery, and health visitors. All this expenditure is subject to annual government budgets, originally set in volume terms, with full allowance for inflation, but limited to a cash figure since the late 1970s. The remaining 21 percent of expenditure relates to general medical services (that is, general practitioners), dentistry, pharmaceutical and ophthalmic services. The majority of the latter expenditures are not subject to budget limits, although for many of these services the patients are required to pay contributory charges, such as for prescriptions, dental treatment and spectacles, and demand is therefore not unlimited.

The effect of these funding arrangements is that governments are able to control more than 80 percent of total health care expenditure and have therefore, since the inception of the NHS in 1948, been able to ensure that it grew in accordance with national economic performance and broad government priorities. Expenditure was restricted in the 1950s, was allowed to grow in the 1960s and 1970s, and has fluctuated in the 1980s. Relative growth has been modest, however, from some 3.5 percent of gross domestic product at inception to rather less than 6 percent at present.

Tight government control of the total amount of expenditure implied by the above has not, however, been extended to control over the nature of the expenditure. The process of allocation of funds is from government to a hierarchy of semi-autonomous statutory health authorities, which are responsible for the actual provision of services within particular localities. Although governments have for some twenty years made statements about priority groups for the expansion of care (broadly the elderly, mentally ill, mentally handicapped, and children), these statements have in the past been mainly hortatory. Haywood and Alaszewski (1980) have demonstrated how the total pattern of health care has amounted to little more than the aggregate of clinical decisions about admission and discharge, diagnosis, and treatment. Official priorities have had limited impact.

A final relevant aspect of NHS structure is the employment status of physicians. Hospital consultants (specialists) as well as junior hospital doctors receive a salary on a scale providing annual increments. In addition the former are allowed to undertake a certain amount of private practice and may receive distinction awards. The latter, which are somewhat unevenly distributed across specializations and geography, are awarded in secret by a committee of the profession on the basis of academic and clinical reputation. There are various grades of award, but the highest approximately doubles the consultant's salary. General medical practitioners are not salaried, but are remunerated largely through NHS capitation fees and practice allowances; they also receive a number of fee-for-service payments for vaccinations and family planning advice.

The effect of these systems of funding and remuneration is to provide relatively little opportunity to increase medical earnings by the performance of additional medical services. Such an increase can only be obtained by consultants engaging in part-time private practice (for which the demand is relatively limited) and by general practitioners either doing the same or increasing the supply of those services for which NHS fees are paid. The logic of the incentives thus created points either towards the maximization of private earnings and/or the pursuit of intellectual or status maximization (perhaps also resulting in a distinction award), or towards the maximization of leisure.

Governments have thus been content to control total NHS spending without controlling its nature. Aaron and Schwartz (1984) have documented the consequent rationing process in which clinicians make individual fragmented and therefore largely invisible decisions both about who shall receive the care available from the limited funds and about the nature of such care. Neither direct patient pressure nor the threat of litigation (much more uncertain for the British plaintiff than the American, who can rely on lawyers' contingency remuneration) has created any significant movements towards peer review of clinical decisions, other than in cases of clinician ill-health.

The lack of government control over the nature and quality of clinical work has been reinforced by a lack of management control, which has arisen from a government guarantee of clinical freedom originally granted in order to ensure medical participation in the NHS upon its creation in 1948 (Willcocks 1967). Hence, management has been officially regarded as a process of facilitating the work of professionals rather than exerting control over them. As recently as 1979, an official document on NHS management arrangements (DHSS 1979) stated

> It is doctors, dentists and nurses and their colleagues in the other health professions who provide the care and cure of patients and promote the health of the people. It is the purpose of management to support them in giving that service.

The above analysis is supported by recent empirical research into the conceptions of clinical freedom held by British consultants and general practitioners (Harrison et al. 1984; Schulz et al. 1985; Pohlman 1985). This research reveals that the respondents regard overall financial limitations as being legitimate restrictions on their autonomy, and indeed a majority accept the principle of individual clinicians being given budgets which may not be exceeded. In sharp contrast, respondents did not see a legitimate role for any mechanism, such as peer review or quality assurance, which restricted their freedom to decide how to treat individual patients. In summary, the nature of clinical autonomy in Britain involves a tight budget within which physicians exercise almost total freedom.

Clinical Autonomy in the United States

Although the medical profession in the United States is usually considered a prime example of an autonomous profession, individual doctors in private practice in the United States generally have less autonomy in their clinical work than their British counterparts in a nationalized health service. On the other hand, while American doctors may have less clinical autonomy, they have had considerably more economic autonomy than British doctors.

Peer surveillance of a doctor's quality of care and use of services has been a long-standing tradition in American hospitals. Unlike Britain, where only specialty trained consultants have hospital admitting and treatment privileges, most licensed physicians in the United States, including general practitioners, seek and usually receive hospital privileges to admit and treat patients. Out of concern for the quality of surgical practices performed by some general practitioners, the American College of Surgeons developed a quality review hospital accreditation programme in the 1920s. In the 1950s this evolved into the Joint Commission on Accreditation of Hospitals (JCAH) which required doctors to evaluate the quality of care of other doctors and to define which procedures individual doctors were qualified to perform in hospitals. In implementing

Medicare and Medicaid in 1966, the federal government essentially adopted this system of accreditation as a criterion for payments to hospitals for federally supported patients. Peer review in American hospital services was further reinforced with the development of professional standards review organizations (PSROs), now called professional review organizations (PROs), whose function is the evaluation of physician hospital care to Medicare patients in order to ensure that the use of services as well as their quality is appropriate. As a result, individual doctors in American hospitals do not have the freedom to treat patients as they wish that is found in British hospitals, but are subject to governance from their hospital medical staff organization and in turn from the hospital board of directors who, ultimately, define what a doctor can and cannot do in hospital.

On the other hand, most doctors in the United States are not salaried employees of any organization as are consultants in the British NHS, nor are they under contract to other organizations as are British GPs. Consequently, as individual entrepreneurs charging the patient (or third-party payer) a fee for the service performed, American doctors have enjoyed more economic autonomy than their NHS counterparts. However, the predominantly fee-for-service (FFS) system in the United States has been a major contributing factor to the rapid rise in health care costs in the United States, which currently approach 11 percent of GNP. Under the FFS system, doctors have financial incentives to provide more services to patients, which enhances physicians' earnings. While such incentives can be in the patients' interests by ensuring that the doctor focuses on patients' needs, they also generate unnecessary services that are not only costly but also possibly hazardous to patients' health. Under the FFS system no one has incentives to contain health care costs except the federal, state and local governments which must meet rising costs from limited taxpayer resources. Approximately 85 percent of the United States population has some health insurance or other means of third-party payment, and most of such schemes cover most hospital charges. Consequently, patients have had few financial incentives not to use their health care benefits. Hospitals, like doctors, have had incentives to attract more patients in order to use more services because as their costs increase so does their income under FFS. Furthermore, until recently, employers, who have paid most employee health care benefits, did not find it difficult to pass on increasing costs in the price of goods sold, and health insurance costs are an attractive tax-free employee benefit under American tax laws.

Widespread patient litigation against doctors has also created an incentive to provide more services to patients. To cover himself or herself should the patient sue, the doctor has an incentive to ensure that all tests and procedures that might conceivably help patients are performed. This is called the practice of defensive medicine. As a result of increasing litigation and awards, malpractice insurance rates have increased sharply, sometimes exceeding $100,000 per physician per annum in more vulnerable specialties in some cities.

The effect of these decentralized forces has been to make difficult any overall control over the system or its costs. The federal government, which pays 29 percent of total national health care costs (state and local government pay another 13 percent) from payroll and general taxes, has generally avoided direct intervention on physician practices. Rather, government controls have centred on hospital costs, which represent 41 percent of total health care costs and have been the fastest-rising component of total health care expenditures. Federal requirements for control over hospital expansion through certificate of need regulations and state hospital rate review controls have only indirectly affected physician behaviour.

In summary, US physicians have accepted restrictions on their clinical autonomy which would be unthinkable to British doctors, but at the same time have had economic autonomy to maximize their earnings. It is also important to note that restrictions on clinical autonomy in the US have heretofore been primarily induced by organized medicine rather than government or other payers. However, payer-induced restrictions are now being rapidly implemented in the United States.

Convergence

One common pressure faced by the health systems of both Britain and the United States has been to contain spending. In both countries, this pressure has become more acute in the last few years, as a result partly of declining national economic performance and partly of government political priorities concerning public expenditure. There are several evident impacts of this pressure upon clinical autonomy.

In Britain, the rate of increase in real NHS expenditure has been falling for some time. It is rather difficult to state a definitive position, because current and capital expenditures are often announced separately and because official statements sometimes quote figures which have been adjusted for notional savings made in efficiency drives. Nevertheless, official sources anticipated a 0.3 percent real reduction for 1985–6, which was of course based on the most favourable method of calculation (*The Guardian*, 18 April 1985). Within this national average, there are quite large geographical variations resulting from policies of resource equalization. Hence, some health authorities face revenue reductions of some significance.

One management reaction, and indeed a political one too, to such cuts is to seek greater efficiency in maximizing outputs from the reduced resource inputs. The initial government strategy was to seek savings in non-clinical areas, and after 1982 various initiatives were launched, including central control of the members of staff not involved in direct patient care, the scrutiny of expenditure in such areas as transport costs and vacancy advertising, and the putting out to private contract of hospital support services such as laundry, cleaning and catering. More recently, partly as a result of the Griffiths report (NHS Management Inquiry 1983) into the management of the service, some other initiatives have been pursued which seem likely to affect clinical autonomy through planning other than global resource constraints on clinical decision-making.

The major initiatives among this latter group are management budgeting, performance indicators, and the prescription blacklist. Management budgeting is a system of control under which expenditure budgets are given to individual clinical decision-makers (or occasionally to groups of them); all expenditure which arises from the decisions, including diagnosis and nursing services, can be charged against such budgets (DHSS 1985). At this level, such budgets do not change the nature of clinical autonomy, but some commentators and managers are proposing a more radical use in order to provide a lever with which to negotiate priority treatment areas with clinicians or to make changes in their practice patterns. Performance indicators are a package of measures of various aspects of NHS activity, which have been developed as means of comparing the relative performance of health authorities. These include a number of indicators which reflect usage of clinical resources, such as lengths of stay within specialties and the turnover of patients per bed per annum (Rathwell and Barnard 1985). It seems more than likely that the revelation of differences in performance in these respects will lead to management pressure for changes in clinician behaviour. Finally, with effect from April 1985, restrictions have been placed upon the hitherto virtually unlimited range of drugs which could be prescribed in the NHS. Some 1,800 substances have been removed from the list of those previously available.

Taken as a whole, these measures mark a significant departure from earlier strategies for expenditure control in that they begin to affect the more detailed processes of clinical decision-making by extending them beyond the individual physician.

In the United States the 1980s have seen dramatic changes in the health environment, with payers facing increasing pressures to control costs and with physicians and other providers becoming vulnerable as a result of excess capacity. With its huge federal deficit, the United States has changed from a creditor nation to one of the largest debtor nations in the world. Health care represents one of the larger and faster-growing contributors to national fiscal problems. Moreover, it is projected that the Medicare system will be bankrupt by the year 1995. To gain control over health care costs, Medicare abandoned FFS hospital payments systems in 1983 and introduced prospective pricing systems (PPS) which pay a flat rate per admission according to 467 diagnostic-related groups (DRGs). The government remains reluctant to intervene directly in physician practices and has applied PPS only to hospital care. However, PPS has reversed the incentives for hospitals in that they will now profit by reducing lengths of stay by Medicare patients and their use of hospital services. Hospital managements, through their medical staff organization, have implemented management information systems and peer utilization review to intervene directly on lengths of stay and utilization practices. Physicians' awareness of practice variations and peer pressures has created a measurable reduction in hospital lengths of stay in general in the United States. While DRGs and associated control systems represent further incursions into individual doctor clinical autonomy, their introduction has largely been made possible by the peer review system which is widely accepted in the United States. Because of the apparent success of DRGs in reducing hospital costs, the federal government is interested in extending them to all Medicare services provided by physicians, although methodological problems as well as doctor opposition have prevented such application to date.

Employers and private insurance carriers, who fund 31 percent of national health care expenditures, have also found rising health care costs intolerable. An example of the burden of health care costs to American industry is the Chrysler Motor Company, which estimated that in 1984 it expended $600 per car or $5,700 per employee for the health care benefits of employees and retired employees, whereas Mitsubishi Motor Company in Japan spent only $374 per employee. Employers in the United States have taken several approaches to containing employee health benefit costs, some of which have also affected physician autonomy. Many employers have placed incentives on employees to reduce utilization of health care by raising deductibles and copayments so that persons using medical services share in the costs. A major Rand Corporation study suggests that through such monetary disincentives utilization and costs can be reduced without adverse affects on an individual's health (Newhouse et al. 1982). Second surgical opinion requirements are another cost containment approach used by employers and a few state Medicaid systems to reduce the numbers of surgical procedures. Second opinion requirements are infringements on doctor autonomy, but the application is consistent with peer review traditions.

Businesses have also formed health care coalitions to increase the power of employers over health care services and costs. Such coalitions provide educational services to employers on ways to intervene on costs by improving employee health as well as by controlling use and prices of services. Business health coalitions and major community employers also contract PROs, which use information systems and physician peer review to monitor employee health care use, costs and quality.

Health maintenance organizations (HMOs) are another employer health care cost control mechanism with a major impact on delivery systems and individual physician autonomy. HMOs are prepaid comprehensive capitation systems with financial incentives to maintain a subscriber's health by using no more services than are absolutely necessary. There are basically three kinds of HMOs: a staff model, whereby physicians are on salary or contract to a consumer- or investor-owned HMO; a group model, whereby a group of physicians owns the HMO; and an independent practice association (IPA), whereby physicians maintain independent practices but contract with the IPA to serve prepaid IPA enrollees and to share in financial risks. Preferred provider organizations (PPOs) are another organizational form intended to promote price competition between health providers. The PPO contracts with doctors to offer a discount to PPO patients. While physicians in PPOs function on an FFS rather than a prepaid basis, discounts presumably facilitate price competition with HMOs. Although they are expanding rapidly, it is important to note that HMOs represented only 7 percent of physician services in the United States in 1984 and PPOs represented even less.

The increasing supply of physicians – a 50,000 physician oversupply is projected by the year 2000 (Bureau of Health Professions 1985) and the increasing competition for patients are forcing doctors into HMOs and PPOs. In order to be competitive, HMOs need to monitor and control use, costs, and presumably quality of services on an out-patient as well as an in-patient basis. While clearly a further infringement of the clinical freedom of individual physicians, it is again achieved through the widely accepted peer review mechanism. Moreover, open competition between plans and monitoring systems along with litigation opportunities increases the power and assertiveness of patients *vis-à-vis* doctors.

Such changes impact not only on the clinical freedom but also on the economic freedom of physicians in the United States. Physician surpluses and competition limit practice location opportunities, and, along with rising expenses such as malpractice insurance, physician earnings are diminishing. While average nominal net income of physicians was nearly $100,000 in 1982, real net income was $40,000, which marks a decline from $41,500 in 1970 (American Medical Association, personal communication). Earnings are likely to continue to decline if competition and HMOs continue to increase. For example, in one city physicians estimate that, owing to price competition, earnings from an HMO patient are only 65 to 70 percent of those from a comparable FFS patient (Schulz and Scheckler 1988).

Concluding Remarks

As a result of these changes in Britain and the United States, a composite picture of potential convergence emerges. Both countries are moving towards greater third-party control of both global health care budgets and clinical decisions. In Alford's terms, these are major challenges by the corporate rationalizer to the dominant professional interests. How the latter will react is a matter for empirical work in the future, but two final observations about the prospects can be made. First, an oversupply of physicians has occurred in the United States; and although the situation is not so clear in Britain, a number of commentators have a similar apprehension. It seems unlikely that such an oversupply will strengthen the profession's position. Secondly, empirical evidence about the attitudes of British physicians towards clinical freedom suggests that in the past at least they have been quick to rationalize occasional breaches (Harrison et al. 1984). The corporate rationalizers seem to be in the ascendant.

10

Structure and Performance of the Medical Care Delivery Systems of the United Kingdom and the United States

J. Rogers Hollingsworth

The central concern of this study is to advance our understanding of why there has been variation in the evolution of the structure of the British and United States medical delivery systems and to shed light on the kinds of performance which have followed from their different structures.

In 1890, the beginning date for the study, hospitals were shunned by those who could afford home care. Medical technology was not very complex, and the tools for medical care were portable enough to fit in the doctor's little black bag. The training of doctors was not very complex, and professional associations were not very active. By 1980, the delivery of medical services had changed markedly in both countries. The British had institutionalized a national health delivery system, with visits to doctors and hospitals 'free' to all and with state coordination important in the development and utilization of research and hospital systems. In contrast, the United States had a medical delivery system with much less state coordination and much more market orientation than that in Britain.

The theoretical perspective for understanding the relationship between the structure and the performance of a medical delivery system is developed here. While the framework is not a theory, it does develop a number of generalizations so that the potential for theory construction is enhanced. In an effort to analyse the variation in the organizational structure, social processes, and performance of the two medical delivery systems, I have relied on two basic theoretical paradigms: an interest-group conflict paradigm, and a social structure paradigm.

This study develops the argument that particular groups both over time and across countries have specific preferences for particular types of system performances, and that the types of performance which get maximized depend on the power of specific groups. In addition, the study attempts to specify the way in which the structure of a delivery system influences the following types of system performance in particular: costs and quality of services, level of innovativeness, equality of access, and standardization across space. For an elaboration of the theoretical position developed here, see Hage and Hollingsworth (1977), Hollingsworth et al. (1978), Hollingsworth and Hanneman (1983) and Hollingsworth (1986).

The Group Conflict Perspective

Over time and across societies, groups differ in their policy preference as to the types of performance desired from various delivery systems. Previously, most research on interest groups has been somewhat idiosyncratic, focusing on specific issues within a single country rather than looking for common themes across time and within and across countries. To overcome this perspective, this study presents a general scheme of interest groups and policy outcomes that applies to most industrialized countries in Western Europe and North America. To make the discussion of interest groups more meaningful, most of the focus is on three major groups which are always relevant: consumers, providers (such as physicians and hospital administrators) and government officials. Consumers are subdivided into lower-income and upper-income groups, as their interests are frequently divergent.

Obviously each of these categories is internally heterogeneous. But for the purposes of explaining (1) investment decisions in medical care, (2) the major decisions concerning access to medical care and the allocation and location of medical resources, and (3) the readiness of systems to adopt various types of change, this strategy does identify the major groups. An analysis of internal group differences is often desirable in order to understand tactical behaviour and short-term phenomena, but unless internal group differences are permanent and deep seated they are relatively unimportant for explaining variations in systems across societies and over long periods (Hage and Hollingsworth 1977; Alford 1975).

Some of the major arguments of the study are sketched in Figure 10.1. Lower-income consumers have tended to be interested in equalizing access to care and benefits via public spending, and in promoting general services rather than highly specialized ones. Upper-income groups have generated pressures for highly indivi- dualized and differentiated services. Thus lower-income consumers have tended to be less concerned than higher-income consumers with innovations, medical research and specialized personal services. Upper-income groups have tended to prefer goods provided by private markets, for the market-place has permitted more pros-

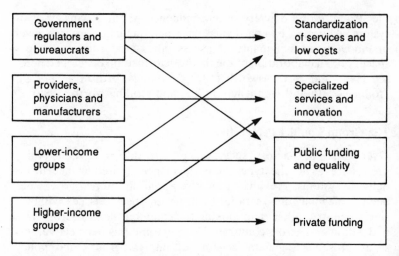

Figure 10.1 *The preferences of various interest groups*

perous individuals to exert influence over the form, quality, and utilization of consumption goods.

For the purposes of this study, there have been two major types of provider influencing system performance: professionals (such as physicians and hospital administrators) and manufacturers. Professional providers have historically attempted to maximize programmatic and technological innovations, since these have called for more development of their special skills and have tended to enhance their incomes and/or prestige. For the same reason, both types of provider have tended to promote the development of specialized services, which in turn have stimulated technical innovations. Because professional providers have tended to prefer the type of organization into which they have been socialized, in both the UK and the US they have been much less inclined to be supportive of organizational innovations – even though the technical innovations which they supported have often led to new types of organization. In both countries, manufacturers (one kind of provider) were not key actors when the level of technological complexity was relatively low. But over time, as technology has become more complex, they have become more influential in bringing about technological innovations, specialized services, and more spending for medical services; and these changes have in turn led to programmatic medical services and organizational changes. Hence, manufacturers since World War II have become key actors in promoting change in the two systems.

Whereas professional providers have often opposed organizational and technological standardization because it usually meant that they would exercise less control over services, government administrators in both countries have tended to favour standardized services as a means of reducing costs and maintaining control over public programmes. For the same reasons, they have been less supportive of technical innovations. Of course, government officials have played an important role in legitimating the entire system in both countries, and as part of this effort they have attempted to coordinate the interests of the other groups. But as the size of the public system has grown, government officials have acquired more autonomy and have had more of an opportunity for their values to shape the system.

Thus there are potentially several natural coalitions. Lower-income groups and government bureaucrats have had some tendency to prefer the same benefits, whereas providers and higher-income groups have had similar preferences. Specifications of the exact lines of cleavage or of coalitions among and between interest groups has varied from case to case, depending on the power of each group at specific times. But the basic distinctions have been among lower- and upper-income consumers, providers, and government administrators, and each of the groups has tended to prefer the types of performance described in Figure 10.1.

The power of interest groups to shape decisions about investments in medical care and about the process of producing medical services has been considerable, and these decisions in turn have shaped the types of performance which have been maximized in the two national delivery systems. The power of groups has not rigidly determined in a mechanistic fashion which performance became maximized, but it has established probabilities that certain tendencies would occur.

Historically, the distribution of power among various groups has tended to give rise to a certain set of institutional arrangements which have shaped the performance of delivery systems, and these arrangements have tended to persist for considerable periods. For this reason, it is important to understand the distribution of power among the key groups of actors at the time that the society first made a major commitment to the widespread distribution of medical technology and the development of a medical delivery system.

Historical generalizations relevant to the relationship between group power and the institutionalization of medical delivery systems are as follows:

1   The more successful lower-income consumers were in shaping

the conditions under which medical services were provided at the time that the society first made a major commitment to the widespread utilization of medical technology, the more the delivery system in its historical evolution emphasized equality in the distribution of and access to medical resources. In the cases of Britain and the United States, there was a sharp difference in the degree to which working men via trade unions and friendly societies organized and entered into contractual relationships with providers.

2   Conversely, the more influential and powerful were the providers at the time the society first made a commitment to the widespread utilization of medical technology, the more inequitable was the distribution of medical resources at subsequent points in time.

3   At the time the society first made a commitment to the widespread utilization of medical technology, the strengths of providers *vis-à-vis* consumers shaped the options for modifying policies at subsequent times, thus limiting the extent to which the two societies were able or willing to modify their delivery systems.

To understand the cross-national variation in medical delivery systems, a historical explanation is necessary because organizations and practices tend to persist once they have been institutionalized and attained legitimacy. Societies have become socialized into different ways of doing things: relationships between clients and providers have become institutionalized, providers have become accustomed to certain forms of payment, and client responses to forms of organisation have become routinized. Of course, organizations and practices of financing medical care which subsequently were unresponsive to popular demands and were based on a technology which clearly became obsolete have suffered losses in legitimacy; when that has occurred, organizations and practices within delivery systems have become substantially modified.

Historically, one of the most important outcomes determined by group power was the form of paying providers. The type of payment across countries has been a key factor in determining whether (1) the system would eventually become predominantly public or private, (2) the system's costs were subject to tight government control or not, (3) it was highly egalitarian with an emphasis on standardized services, (4) it was highly innovative, and (5) it tended to place high or low emphasis on very specialized services.

By knowing which interest groups have the most power early in a system's history, one can make predictions about which funding outcomes were most likely to evolve in the history of a national medical delivery system. The greater the power of professional providers *vis-à-vis* consumers, the greater the likelihood that payments would eventually become indirect (government or insurance company paying the consumer, who, in turn, would pay the providers), thus removing the provider from the control of the government or other insurer. The greater the power of the consumer *vis-à-vis* the professional provider, the greater the likelihood that payments would become direct (government or insurance company paying the professional provider), thus subjecting the provider to greater controls of the paying authority. Historically the more control the government or other insurers have exercised over the provider, the less costly and less innovative the system. Moreover, the more extensive the public funding, the more equitable the access to delivery systems; conversely, when payments have been privately financed, there has been greater inequality in access to medical care (Abel-Smith 1965; Hogarth 1963; Glaser 1970).

The group conflict perspective developed in this study argues that groups systematically have different preferences, and that the distribution of power among groups in the United Kingdom and the United States during the late nineteenth and early twentieth century influenced the medical payment mechanism. The choices about payment mechanisms carried significant consequences for system performances such as equality of access, costs, innovativeness, and standardization in spatial terms.

The Structural Perspective: the Problem of Centralization

The power of groups is only one type of variable which has shaped the history and the performance of the two delivery systems. Another key variable has been centralization. This is an important factor which has too long been ignored in the social science literature, for it has a significant impact on the performance of national delivery systems. Irrespective of which group has dominated the system, centralization has placed constraints on system performance. For example, increasing the level of centralization has led to more public spending and generalized services, greater equality among social classes and groups, and more cost controls and standardization. Decentralization has led to specialized services, diversity of services among different groups, and technical innovations (Hollingsworth and Hanneman 1983; Hage and Hollingsworth 1977).

By centralization is meant the level at which strategic decisions are made about personnel, budgets, programmes and standards. A delivery system in which all of these decisions have been made in the private sector has been more decentralized than one in which the decisions have been made in the public sector. And in the public sector, a delivery system in which all decisions have been made by local authorities has been less centralized than one in which the decisions have been made at the national level. In reality, however, all strategic decisions have rarely been made at one level. In the United States, for example, there has been much private as well as public decision-making about medical care at all levels of the society (local, state and federal).

Too often, scholars have referred to a society as being highly centralized, when in fact within the same society it has been possible for the medical delivery system to be decentralized. Moreover, the level of centralization is constantly changing in all systems. It is desirable that we be mindful of this fact and that we attempt to understand how performances have changed in response to changes in the level of centralization.

Centralized systems have tended to opt for standardized programmes and services for different groups and in different parts of a country; thus under certain conditions, centralized systems have had greater potential for cutting costs. Historically, the major advantage of a more centralized system has been that it has allowed considerable rationalization of service delivery. It has been able to provide essentially the same service to all and at lower costs. Increases in the level of centralization have tended to bring about more standardization across regions, more effective cost controls, and greater equality to services among social classes and groups. Thus, there have been trade-offs among performances. Systems which have been very egalitarian have had fewer specialized and individualized services. Those which have engaged in effective cost controls have been reluctant to adopt new innovations (see Figure 10.2).

Across countries, centralized systems have been less costly in financial terms, but they have tended to be less innovative. There has been much literature which indicates that centralization has stifled the adoption of new ideas and slowed down the process of communication (Hollingsworth et al. 1978; Ben-David 1960; Hage 1980; Aiken and Hage 1971).

Even though centralization has acted as a constraint on the costs and the innovativeness of medical delivery systems, it is important to note that historically the costs and the level of innovativeness have been increased within each country as its medical delivery system has become more centralized. As societies have acquired

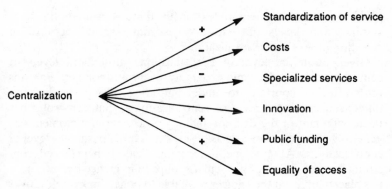

Figure 10.2   *Relationships between centralization and performance*

more wealth per capita in the process of economic development, they have spent more, and by spending more, they have become more innovative. The argument here is that after controlling for wealth and other variables which influence costs and innovativeness, centralized systems have been less innovative and have spent less money than decentralized systems.

In highly centralized systems, the costs of changing standards become considerable. And historically reluctance to take action has increased with the cost. Under these circumstances, inertia occurred and providers found it difficult to develop programme innovations. Moreover, decision-makers in centralized systems were unlikely to be aware of problems throughout the society and therefore did not perceive the need for change until there was mounting unrest and pressure from particular interest groups.

Publicly financed delivery systems have provided greater equality of access to services among social classes and groups than have privately financed ones. These publicly financed systems have usually been more centralized. Thus it appears that greater centralization has led to greater equality of access to services among classes and groups.

Interaction between Centralization and Interest Groups

It is one thing to comprehend how variation in group power and in the level of centralization has influenced the performance of medical delivery systems, but it is much more difficult to specify the interaction between group power and the level of centralization. It is important to point out that irrespective of what group has dominated a delivery system, the level of centralization has had predictable consequences on the system's performance. For example, providers have been more powerful than consumers in both systems, but levels of innovativeness have varied because of variation in levels of centralization.

Given an initial level of centralization, subsequent levels of centralization are determined largely by group conflict. For this reason it is important to understand how group conflict has influenced the initial level of centralization. Whatever group has been dominant in the decision-making process at any moment has generally wanted to keep decision-making at that particular level of centralization. At any one time, centralization has placed constraints on the ability of particular groups to influence policy, and it has placed limits on the choices available to policy-makers. But over long periods, the power of groups and group conflict have changed the levels of centralization in both systems.

Historically, those who have believed that they are unable to change policies in the decision-making process have usually wanted to increase the level of centralization as a means of increasing their power, even though a higher level of centralization has often placed constraints on the types of utilities which they have preferred. In an effort to standardize resources in spatial terms and to equalize access to services, lower-income groups have usually attempted to shift decision-making to a more centralized level. As medical technology has been perceived as being efficacious, complex, and expensive, low-income consumers have historically turned to the government for assistance in providing medical care. As lower-income groups have mobilized their power and demanded medical services, most medical delivery systems have become more centralized over time.

On the other hand providers, on a few occasions, have preferred decision-making at a national level, particularly when they have believed that they could mobilize power and operate effectively at that level. This was the case in 1948 when the British consultants preferred to be employed by the national rather than the local government because they believed they would have more influence at the national level. In an effort to shape decisions, professional providers have usually had an advantage over lower-income consumers in mobilizing power at the central level. The degree to which a group has been able to organize effectively at the national level has depended on the total resources of the group. Resources have consisted of the size of the group as well as such per capita resources as money, education, and status. Because physicians have had high per capita resources, over time they have generally had more success than consumer organizations in mobilizing political power at the national level, even though consumers may initially have been responsible for the system's becoming centralized. Moreover, providers have historically had an advantage in maximizing political power because they have usually belonged to a single-issue organization and have been able to focus all of their energies on the one policy area with which they were concerned. In contrast, most consumer organizations (such as labour unions) have been multi-issue organizations with their energies diffused among many policy areas. Relative to providers, consumers on a per capita basis have usually had lower status, less money, and less education, thus restricting their ability to mobilize power at the central level.

Thus there is a certain irony in the historical relationship between the participation of interest groups and increasing centralization. It has been the weakness of consumer groups *vis-à-vis* providers that has led consumer groups to demand higher levels of decision-making. Consumers have usually been the catalyst in increasing the level of the decision-making process, because they generally believed that decision-making at higher levels would enhance their interests. As centralization increased, however, the balance of power to influence decisions has tended to remain decidedly in favour of providers.

The capacity of consumers to *create* decision-making authorities at higher levels of society by the mobilization of votes has tended to be far greater than the capacity to *control* such units once they have been created. This has occurred because of the limited and indirect representation of groups in the decision-making process at higher levels of society.

The relationship between centralization and the degree of participation has been a complex one. At the most simple level, the shift of decision-making to higher levels of society has generally been a direct consequence of increased participation by previously excluded groups. In turn, higher levels of decision-making have usually accomplished the intended purpose of broadening participation, at least initially. However, the shift to a higher level of decision-making has altered the manner in which groups have been represented and has created new and powerful interest groups, often leading to a decline in the level of direct participation by the groups that were responsible for the change in the level of decision-making.

On the other hand, consumers have had one potential advantage over providers – their numerical superiority. Across countries, when consumers have been able to develop an encompassing organization (such as one that encompasses a substantial percentage of the society's total population), they have been able to exercise considerable influence over the decision-making process at the national level. But whether consumers have been able to get organized at a national level in this fashion has depended on several variables. Consumers have had greater potential to develop encompassing organizations when the country has been smaller, the society more homogeneous ethnically and linguistically, and the economy less complex and diverse. Hence, consumers in countries such as Norway and Sweden have had considerable capacity for the development of encompassing group formation. Because the United States historically has been a large, multicultural society with a complex economy, consumers there have had low capacity for developing encompassing organizations and mobilizing consumer power at the local or national level. Thus providers have not had too much difficulty in dominating the decision-making process in America. The United Kingdom historically has fallen midway between the Scandinavian and American cases in the ability of consumers (especially lower-income consumers) to develop encompassing groups and to mobilize their power (Hollingsworth 1982). Of course professional providers have been powerful in the medical delivery systems of all highly industrialized societies. What is variable has been their power *vis-à-vis* consumers.

Over time, medical delivery systems have had multiple levels of authority in highly industrialized societies. In both the UK and the US there has been an incremental shift towards multiple levels of authority, and there has been a persistence of decision-making authorities at lower levels of delivery systems – a persistence which is not difficult to understand from the interest-group perspective. Each new level of decision-making authority has developed a set of officials and constituencies to participate in the decision-making process. Thus there have been interest groups organized to participate at each level of decision-making. Over time, decision-making authorities have proliferated, each permitting the participation of various interest groups. Partly as a result of this proliferation, the administrative machinery of both delivery systems has become increasingly complex. And while consumer groups have played an important role in promoting a more centralized decision-making process, it has been providers as well as public officials and administrators who have become the dominant actors in the decision-making process. While multilevel systems appear to be effective in broadening the scope of group participation, groups with high levels of organizational capacities and specialized knowledge have become more successful in influencing decision-making in centralized delivery systems.

Determinants of Group Power and Centralization

Many factors influence the power of groups and the level of centralization of the UK and US delivery systems, but there are four variables which consistently across the two societies and over time have placed limits on the power of groups and the level of centralization: size, social heterogeneity, technology, and wealth.

Size
Among social services delivery systems in democratic societies, those in large societies have been somewhat more decentralized than those in smaller societies (Hollingsworth and Hanneman 1983). Of course, size does not constrain centralization in some mechanistic fashion. But larger societies have more levels of hierarchy and more parts to be coordinated, and these place constraints on how centralized a system may become. Hence, all other things being equal, one would expect a democratic country the size of the United States to have a medical delivery system somewhat more decentralized than that in Britain.

Even though the size of the country in a cross-national perspective has been inversely correlated with the level of centralization in the two systems, the relationship has been just the opposite when viewed historically within the two countries. Throughout the twentieth century, the medical delivery systems of these two countries have increased in size as a result of expansion in the numbers of physicians, nurses, para-professionals, hospital beds and so on. At the same time, both medical delivery systems have become more centralized, as low-income groups have demanded that governments play a larger role in providing medical services. Hence, within the two countries, increases in the size of medical delivery systems and centralization have tended to trend in the same direction, though these trends are not causally related. But even if the power of low-income consumers has been an important reason why medical delivery systems have become more centralized over time, medical delivery systems in larger societies have tended to be more decentralized than those in smaller societies; the larger the country, the more difficult it has been for low-income consumers to mobilize and organize sufficient power to change the structure of the delivery system.

Social heterogeneity
As suggested above, because American society has been more heterogeneous ethnically, radically, and religiously, the lines of cleavage among consumer groups have been very sharp. For this

reason, it has been difficult for low-income consumers to develop organizations powerful enough to dominate the medical delivery system. Because of the fragmented power of American consumer groups, they have historically not been very successful in marshalling the power necessary to bring about a highly centralized delivery system. Conversely, because American society has had greater social heterogeneity than Britain, professional providers *vis-à-vis* consumers have exercised greater power in shaping the performance of the American system.

Technology

The technology of all medical delivery systems has become more differentiated and complex during the twentieth century. As the technology has become more complex, professional providers and others with expertise have become more influential *vis-à-vis* consumers in shaping decisions about the nature of medical investments and the production of medical services – irrespective of the level of centralization. Hence providers in the American as well as in the British medical delivery systems have become increasingly more influential during the twentieth century. However, the historical record demonstrates that medical delivery systems which are decentralized and which are dominated by professional providers have been more receptive to new and expensive technology than those which have been relatively centralized and which have been dominated by low-income consumers.

Systems which historically have been dominated by providers and have been quite decentralized have tended to be very receptive to highly complex technology and to become increasingly autonomous as a result of high levels of technological complexity. As medical technology has become more complex and specialized, it has become more difficult for any group to dominate and to manage the system. Moreover, no group in either the US or the UK has been able to assess the technological needs of the society. As a result, technology has tended to develop a logic of its own, with specialization begetting higher and higher levels of specialization. Therefore there has been a tendency in both countries to err on the side of expanding the system, spending more money, and developing alternative but even more complex technologies. In both countries, the systems have dictated much of their own demands, and they have shaped the thinking of the entire society about the type of technology needed in order to achieve good health. As the technology has become highly specialized, the policy debates about system characteristics have become more and more restricted. Knowledge of the activities and behaviour of the whole system has become increasingly irrelevant for policy decisions. Policy-makers have tended to consider only those decisions whose known consequences have differed marginally from the status quo. In both countries, it has become increasingly difficult for anyone to understand fully the entire medical delivery system, because of its high degree of complexity. Since decisions have been made primarily about specialized parts, but not the whole of the system, the system in each country has threatened to take on a life of its own as it has become increasingly immune to conscious interference from groups in its environment. Devoid of any clear vision of purpose, the two systems have increasingly been shaped by an unfolding of the logic of technological imperatives. Because the British system has historically been more centralized and subject to more popular control, it has tended to be more resistant to the absorption of new and more complex technology than the American system. Moreover, the British system has remained somewhat less autonomous.

As long as highly specialized systems have produced relatively satisfactory results, they have posed no serious problems. But highly complex medical systems tend to become increasingly costly, causing the society eventually to face a crisis over the costs of medical care; this has been the case in America. Because the very structure of the system has been largely responsible for the crisis, American society appears to have had little capacity to cope with the crisis. On the other hand, the centralized British system, which historically has been more subject to popular control and has been less permeable to high technology, has tended to remain somewhat more immune to the crisis of rising medical costs.

Wealth

Like the previous variables, the effect of wealth on the level of centralization and the power of groups in the two systems has been indirect. Its effects have been mediated by its impact on the state and its revenue system. As the gross national product has risen in the UK and the US, these countries have tended to change their revenue system, with an increasing share of the revenue being raised by an income tax. Most income taxes have been raised primarily at the central levels of government, and governments have had a tendency to formulate and implement policy at the level at which revenues have been collected. Hence, as more and more revenues have been collected at the central level of government, more functions (such as medical services) have historically been shifted to the central level. Meantime, technology has become more complex with the expansion of a society's wealth; as low-income consumers have demanded that government make the technology available to them, the central government has responded by making medical resources available with funding at the level at which revenues have been collected.

At some point in the economic development of both societies, the governmental sector began to expand more rapidly than the economy. And in both societies, it was the governmental sector at central rather than local level which began to grow most rapidly – meaning that both medical delivery systems tended to become more centralized as GNP expanded. Because those with specialized knowledge tended to operate more efficiently at centralized levels than did low-income consumers, this process has tended to enhance the power of specialized providers in shaping decisions about the production of medical care.

Variation in System Performance

Because the two systems have differed so much in their distribution of power and levels of centralization, they have performed very differently in terms of access to care, costs, innovativeness, and quality of care.

Equality
Both systems have become more egalitarian in access to medical care over time, but in respect to most medical technology the British system has remained much more egalitarian. In both countries, low-income consumers now visit physicians more frequently than do those with upper incomes. But in both countries, the physician spends more time with upper-income consumers when there is a consultation and is more knowledgeable about their problems. Moreover, there is evidence that upper-income groups receive somewhat higher quality of care in both countries (Goodman 1980b; Cartwright and O'Brien 1976; LeGrand 1978). Why this occurs is not entirely clear, but upper-income groups in both countries ask doctors more questions and provide more information.

But a critical difference in the two countries is that approximately 35 million Americans are still not covered by private medical insurance or by government Medicaid and Medicare. Approximately 70 percent of these uninsured people are low-income individuals who are effectively priced out of the medical care market. In the more market-oriented American system, prices limit the quantity of goods and services which are available for millions of other Americans, thus acting as a deterrent to the consumption of medical services. On the other hand, even though money prices have been abolished in the UK National Health Service, waiting lists act as a deterrent to the consumption of services. While waiting lists do not have a systematic bias against low-income consumers, upper-income consumers may jump the queue by purchasing care in the private market.

In both countries, there is still an inadequate relationship between the need for medical services and the distribution of medical resources. In both countries, medical resources are least adequate in the areas which need it most. British scholars have demonstrated considerable variation in the regional distribution of medical resources; those regions which were well endowed with resources at the start of the National Health Service have tended to retain their advantages. However, regional variation in the distribution of resources has narrowed much more rapidly in Britain than in the United States, and most medical resources have been more equitably distributed across regions in Britain than in America.

Costs

For some years the system in Britain has spent about one-half as much per person on medical care as the American system. Moreover, the British have spent a much smaller percentage of their gross national product on medical care than the Americans. It is true that as per capita income rises in a country, the percentage of the GNP which it spends on medical care also rises. Because Britain's per capita income is lower than that in America, it would be expected to spend a smaller share of its GNP on medical care.

However, the organization of the medical delivery system is a key variable in constraining medical expenditures. The American method of payment on a fee-for-service basis combined with a retrospective reimbursement scheme has encouraged a medical delivery system which has had little incentive for economy. Indeed, the American system has rewarded providers of care for cost-increasing behaviour. In Britain, however, the government has effectively used its monopoly power to keep medical costs low. The British have paid less for drugs than have the citizens of any other country in Western Europe and North America (Cooper and Cooper 1972; Goodman 1980a); and by American and European standards, the salaries of British doctors have been quite low for more than a quarter of a century. While one has heard more complaints among young doctors in training in Britain than in America, surveys of the British medical profession have consistently reported the morale of the medical profession to be quite high (Culyer et al. 1980). In America, in order to differentiate themselves from their peers and to appear to be practising high-quality medicine, doctors have insisted on and have generally received the best and most expensive medical technology available. In Britain, however, physicians have been less influential and the system has tended to demonstrate a preference for routine and less expensive treatment strategies.

There appears to be some basis for concluding that the fee-for-service system operating in America has encouraged doctors to carry out more medical procedures than their counterparts in the National Health Service. On the other hand, some analysts have argued that the NHS system of paying practitioners on a capitation basis has encouraged them to prefer the trivial to the non-trivial case and to over-refer patients to hospital-based doctors (Glaser 1970; Goodman 1980a: 63). While there is some justification for this perspective, the British general practitioner has had an incentive to convince those on his lists that he is looking after their best interests; otherwise they would gravitate to another practitioner.

Innovativeness
This study has suggested that while centralized systems tend to constrain the level of expenditures on medical care, centralization has placed constraints on the adoption of new ideas and slowed down the diffusion of complex and expansive technologies. Centralization has slowed down the diffusion process because certain groups which have preferred innovativeness have been less involved in the decision-making process. Moreover, centralization has meant that there has been greater reliance on public funding. In centralized systems, government bureaucrats have been more involved in the decision-making process, and they, more than private entrepreneurs, have tended to perceive certain types of innovations as costly and unnecessary.

Throughout the twentieth century, the British system has been relatively inventive. However, the evidence is somewhat mixed concerning the diffusion of innovations. Following 1962, when the regulation of new drugs was more centralized and rigorous in America than in Britain, new drugs tended to diffuse more slowly in America. But over time there has been convergence in the diffusion of new drugs in the two countries, as the British regulatory system has adopted most of the American guidelines for testing the safety and efficacy of new drugs.

On the other hand, the centralized and cost-conscious UK National Health Service has been much slower to adopt expensive new technologies. For example Britain, consistent with its inventiveness, was the country where much of the technology for the full-body scanner was developed. But at late as 1976 there were fewer than 25 brain scanners and only four full-body scanners in use in the whole UK. In the United States at the same time, however, there were more than 1,000 in use – over half of which were produced in Britain (Goodman 1980a).

Again, the British were pioneers in the development of renal dialysis technology. But in 1976 the National Health Service accepted only one-half as many new patients per 1,000,000 population as most West European countries. At the same time that the British were treating 7.1 patients per 100,000 with dialysis, the United States was treating 12 per 100,000. Meantime, the British have also made much less frequent use of open-heart surgery and other expensive technologies – the efficaciousness of which have often been open to question. In sum, the British have placed much less emphasis on non-routine and expensive technology than have the Americans, who by the middle 1970s had what many medical economists considered to be an excess of hospital capacity in every metropolitan area. Indeed, the United States had such a surplus of surgeons that most carried substantially less than a full workload (Fuchs 1979).

Quality of care
While almost every student of medical care is interested in assessing the quality of patient care, most scholars have little choice but to acknowledge the difficulty of operationalizing that concept. By definition, quality is concerned with the effect of care on the health of individuals. Though numerous researchers have attempted to develop an index of the quality of hospital care, thus far there has been very little attention devoted to assessing the quality of national medical delivery systems. While at a high level of abstraction it is possible to compare almost anything, it is very difficult (though important) to compare the overall quality of care in Britain with that in America because the two systems have attempted to do quite different things. American practitioners during the twentieth century have been more concerned with diagnosing and treating sickness, while their counterparts in Britain have been more concerned with helping individuals to cope with their everyday work situations. Using a wide variety of laboratory tests, American physicians have tended to examine their patients more frequently and thoroughly for physical disease, while British doctors have tended to be more concerned with helping patients to deal with a variety of anxiety states and to cope with the stresses of everyday life. As Rosemary Stevens suggests, modern technology has 'been incorporated into the systems of each country in different ways, reflecting pre-existing patterns of professional development and

social attitudes toward the provision of care' (Stevens 1976: 28).

The most frequent complaint heard in and out of Britain about the quality of care provided by the NHS has focused on the long waiting lists for hospital care. Certainly this subject is complex. As a percentage of patients receiving hospital care, waiting lists have not increased in Britain over time. Moreover, waiting lists usually contain the names of some patients who have already been cured, who have moved, or who have died. However, econometric studies have demonstrated that increasing the supply of physicians and hospital beds has had little effect in reducing the size of waiting lists. Rather, increasing the supply of doctors and hospital beds has encouraged general practitioners to refer more patients to hospitals and hospital-based doctors to assign patients to waiting lists (Feldstein 1967; Culyer 1976; Klein 1983a). In short, waiting lists constitute a poor indicator for the quality of care provided by the NHS.

The Americans have excelled in the development of centres containing modern and expensive technology for the diagnosis and treatment of disease. For upper-income groups, there may be no better diagnostic and treatment centres in the world. On the other hand, the services provided by the National Health Service for low-income patients are probably better than those provided by the American system for its low-income citizens. Those who can afford the best in Britain have often complained about the inadequacies of the system, while low-income citizens have been very grateful for the type of services which have been available (Culyer 1976). In America, there has been much greater variation in the type of care received by the poor and the better-off than in Britain. Moreover, many Americans (especially the poor) have had inadequate access to high-quality medical care, a phenomenon which disappeared in Britain with the adoption of the NHS.

The record suggests that there have been trade-offs among certain performances. For example, there has been a trade-off between a widespread commitment to equality of access to care and the rapid diffusion of new, expensive medical technology. Moreover, this type of trade-off has occasionally compromised the principle of equality. The UK has had a much stronger commitment to equality than the United States; and to achieve this goal, the British have developed a highly centralized system in which government officials have been very cost conscious. In the process they have encountered fundamental tensions between the performance of low costs and equality of access to expensive new technology.

The history of these two systems suggests that the system which opts to have very expensive and highly specialized services is likely to have many centres which dispense very high-quality services but which only upper-income groups can easily afford. On the other hand, the system which attempts to meet the minimum needs of all of its citizens – as the British system has done – will emphasize routine care, less expensive treatment strategies, and less specialized services.

Note

I wish to thank my colleagues Robert Hanneman and Jerald Hage for some insights reflected in this chapter.

References

Aaron, H.J. and Schwartz, W.B. (1984) *The Painful Prescription*. Washington, DC: Brookings Institution.

Abel-Smith, Brian (1965) The Major Pattern of Financing and the Organization of Medical Services that have Emerged in Other Countries. *Medical Care*, 3: 33–40.

Abernethy, D.S. and Pearson, David A. (1979) *Regulating Hospital Costs: the Development of Public Policy*. Ann Arbor, MI: AUPHA Press.

Aiken, Michael and Hage, Jerry (1971) The Organic Organization and Innovation. *Sociology*, 5: 63–82.

Alford, Robert R. (1975) *Health Care Politics: Ideological and Interest Group Barriers to Reform*. Chicago: University of Chicago Press.

Altenstetter, Christa (1974) *Health Policy-Making and Administration in West Germany and the United States*. Beverly Hills, CA: Sage.

Altenstetter, Christa (1980) Hospital Planning in France and the Federal Republic of Germany. *Journal of Health Politics, Policy and Law*, 5: 309–32.

Altenstetter, Christa (1982) Ziele, Instrumente und Widersprüchlichkeiten der Deutschen Krankenhauspolitik, Vergleichend Dargestellt am Beispiel der Bundespflegesatzverordnung. Wissenschaftszentrum, Berlin, report P/82-2.

Altenstetter, Christa (1985a) *Krankenhausbedarfsplanung*. Munich: Oldenbourg.

Altenstetter, Christa (1985b) Hospital Policy and Resource Allocation in the Federal Republic of Germany 1972–1983. In Groth and Wade 1985: 237–65.

Altenstetter, Christa (1985c) Hospital Planning and Regulation in Germany: 1945–1984. *Proceedings of the XIIIth World Congress of the International Political Science Association*, Paris.

Altenstetter, Christa (1986a) German Social Security Programs: an Interpretation of their Development, 1883–1983. In Ashford and Kelley 1986: 73–97.

Altenstetter, Christa (1986b) Reimbursement Policy of Hospitals in the Federal Republic of Germany. *International Journal of Health Planning and Management*, 1(3): 189–211.

Altenstetter, Christa and Björkman, James Warner (1978) *Federal State Health Policies and Impacts: the Politics of Implementation*. Washington, DC: University Press of America.

Altenstetter, Christa and Björkman, James Warner (1981) Planning and Implementation: a Comparative Perspective on Health Policy. *International Political Science Review*, 2: 11–42.

Anderson, John E. (ed.) (1976) *Cases in Public Policy Making*. New York: Praeger.

Anderson, Odin W. and Shields, M. (1982) Quality Measurement and Control in Physician Decision Making: State of the Art. *Health Services Research*, 2: 125–55.

Ascoli, U. (ed.) (1984) *Welfare State all'Italiana*. Bari: Laterza.

Ashford, Douglas E. (ed.) (1978a) *Comparing Public Policy: New Concepts and Methods*. Beverly Hills, CA: Sage.

Ashford, Douglas E. (1978b) Structural Analysis of Policy, or Institutions Do Matter. In Ashford 1978a: 81–98.

Ashford, Douglas E. and Kelley, E.W. (eds) (1986) *Nationalizing Social Security in Europe and America*. Greenwich, CT: JAI Press.

Averyt, William F., Björkman, James Warner and Foltz, Anne-Marie (1976) *Medical Societies and the Struggle over Fee Systems in Medicare and Medicaid.* New Haven: Yale School of Medicine.

Badura, B. and von Ferber, C. (1981) *Selbsthilfe und Selbstorganisation im Gesundheitswesen.* Munich: Oldenbourg.

Badura, B. and von Ferber, C. (1983) *Laienpotential: Patientenaktivierung und Gesundheitsselbsthilfe.* Munich: Oldenbourg.

Baier, H. (1978) *Medizin im Sozialstaat.* Stuttgart: Fritz Enke.

Barnard, Keith and Lee, Kenneth (eds) (1977) *Conflicts in the National Health Service.* London: Croom Helm.

Barral, E. (1978) *Economie de la santé: faits et chiffres.* Paris: Dunod.

Beer, Samuel H. (1978) Federalism, Nationalism and Democracy in America. *American Political Science Review,* 72: 400–31.

Behrends, B. (1983) Die Entwicklung der Rechtsprechung zum Pflegesatzrecht nach dem Krankenhausfinanzierungsgesetz und der Bundespflegesatzverordnung. *Die Ortskrankenkasse,* 14–15: 640–9.

Ben-David, J. (1960) Scientific Productivity and Academic Organization in Nineteenth Century Medicine. *American Sociological Review,* 25: 828–43.

Berlant, Jeffrey (1975) *Profession and Monopoly: a Study of Medicine in the United States and Great Britain.* Berkeley, CA: University of California Press.

Berlinguer, G. (1973) *Medicina e Politica.* Bari: De Donato.

Berlinguer, G. (1979) *Una Riforma per la Salute.* Bari: De Donato.

Björck, Gunnar (1977) How to be a Clinician in a Socialist Country. *Annals of Internal Medicine,* 86: 813–17.

Björkman, James Warner (1982) Professionalism in the Welfare State: Sociological Saviour or Political Pariah? *European Journal of Political Research,* 10: 407–28.

Björkman, James Warner (1985a) Who Governs the Health Sector? Comparative European and American Experiences with Representation, Participation and Decentralization. *Comparative Politics,* 17: 399–420.

Björkman, James Warner (1985b) Health Policy and Politics in Sri Lanka: Developments in the South Asian Welfare State. *Asian Survey,* 25: 537–52.

Björkman, James Warner (1986) Health Policy and Human Capital: the Case of Pakistan. *Pakistan Development Review,* 25: 281–330.

Björkman, James Warner and Altenstetter, Christa (1979) Accountability in Health Care: an Essay on Mechanisms, Muddles and Mires. *Journal of Health Politics, Policy and Law,* 4: 360–81.

Björkman, James Warner and Silver, George A. (1978) Citizen Control of Health Services: an International Perspective on Participation, Representation and Social Policy. *Proceedings of the IXth World Congress of Sociology,* Uppsala.

Bjurulf, Bo and Swahn, Urban (1980) Health Policy Recommendations and What Happened to Them: Sampling the 20th Century Record. In Heidenheimer and Elvander 1980: 75–98.

Blumstein, J. (1976) Inflation and Quality: the Case of PSROs. In Zubkoff 1976: 246–73.

Bogs, H. and von Ferber, C. (eds) (1978) *Soziale Selbstverwaltung.* Bonn: Verlag der Ortskrankenkassen.

Bompiani, A. (1984) La Formazione del Medico. In Freddi 1984a: 119–56.

Bonß, W. and Riedmüller, B. (1982) Verbands- und Kommunalpolitik: zum Verhältnis von staatlicher und außerstaatlicher Psychiatriepolitik. In Keupp and Rerrich 1982: 107–16.

Boulanger, W. (1984) Editorial. *Wisconsin Medical Journal,* 83: 6.

Brenna, A. (ed.) (1984) *Il Governo della Spesa Sanitaria*. Rome: Servizio Italiano Pubblicazioni Internazionali.

Brown, Larry D. (1983) Common Sense Meets Implementation: Certificate of Need Regulation in the States. *Journal of Health Politics, Policy and Law*, 8: 480–94.

Bruckenberger, E. (1985) Medizinisch-technische Großgeräte: diagnostischer Overkill und das niedersächsische Kooperationsmodell. *Deutsches Ärzteblatt*, 30: 2175–8.

Bundesminister für Arbeit und Sozialordnung (1985) *Die Gesetzliche Krankenversicherung in der Bundesrepublik Deutschland im Jahre 1983*. Bonn.

Bungener, Martine (1984) Une Eternelle Pléthore médicale? *Sciences Sociales et Santé*, 2 (février): 77–110.

Bureau of Health Professions (1985) *Projections of Physician Supply in the US*. Rockville, MD: BHP.

Cairns, J.A. and Snell, M.C. (1978) Prices and the Demand for Care. In Culyer and Wright 1978: 95–122.

Cannegieter, D. (1954) *Honderdvijftig Jaar Gezondheidswet*. Assen: Van Gorcum.

Carder, Max and Klingeberg, Bendix (1980) Towards a Salaried Medical Profession: How 'Swedish' was the Seven Crowns Reform? In Heidenheimer and Elvander 1980: 143–72.

Carels, E.J., Neuhauser, Duncan and Stason, W.B. (eds) (1980) *The Physician and Cost Control*. Cambridge, MA: Oelschlager, Gunn and Hain.

Cartwright, A. and O'Brien, M. (1976) Social Class Variations in Health Care and in the Nature of General Practitioner Consultations. In Stacey 1976: 77–98.

Castles, F.G. and Wildemann, Rudolf (eds) (1986) *Visions and Realities of Party Government*. Berlin, New York: de Gruyter.

Cavazzuti, F. and Giannini, S. (1982) *La Riforma Malata*. Bologna: Il Mulino.

Charles, C.A. (1976) The Medical Profession and Health Insurance: an Ontario Case Study. *Social Science and Medicine*, 10: 33–8.

Checkoway, B. (ed.) (1981) *Citizens and Health Care*. New York: Pergamon.

Chubb, J.E. (1983) *Interest Groups and the Bureaucracy: the Politics of Energy*. Stanford, CA: Stanford University Press.

Cleverly, William (ed.) (1982) *Handbook of Health Care Accounting and Finance*. Rockville, MD: Aspen.

Collins, Doreen (1969) The French Social Security Reform of 1967. *Public Administration*, 1: 91–111.

Commissie Structuuren Financiering Gezondheidszorg (1987) *Bereidheid tot verandering*. Den Haag: Staatsuitgeverij.

Cooper, M.H. and Cooper, A.J. (1972) *International Price Comparisons: a Study of the Prices of Pharmaceuticals in the United Kingdom and Eight Other Countries*. London: National Economic Development Office.

Coser, R.L. (1958) Authority and Decision Making in a Hospital. *American Sociological Review*, 23: 54–64.

Covell, R. (1980) The Impact of Regulation of Health Care Quality. In Levin 1980: 111–25.

Crozier, Michel (1964) *The Bureaucratic Phenomenon*. Chicago: University of Chicago Press.

Crozier, Michel (1986) Perché il Gioco è una Metafora più Utile per la Ricerca Organizzativa. In Sacconi 1986: 199–225.

Culyer, A.J. (1976) *Need and the National Health Service*. London: Martin Robertson.

Culyer, A.J. and Wright, K.G. (eds) (1978) *Economic Aspects of Health Services*. London: Martin Robertson.

Culyer, A.J., Maynard, A. and Williams, A. (1980) An Essay on Motes and Beams: an Appraisal of Alternative Mechanisms for the Provision of Health Care. Paper presented at the Conference on Health Care sponsored by the American Enterprise Institute, Washington, DC.

Dahl, Robert (1961) *Who Governs? Democracy in an American City*. New Haven, CT: Yale University Press.

Dahl, Robert (1984) *Modern Political Analysis*. 4th edn. Englewood Cliffs, NJ: Prentice-Hall.

Delogu, S. (1967) *Sanità Pubblica. Sicurezza Sociale e Programmazione Economica*. Turin: Centro di Ricerca e Documentazione Luigi Einaudi.

Deppe, H.U. (ed.) (1983) *Gesundheitssysteme und Gesundheitspolitik in Westeuropa*. Frankfurt-am-Main, New York: Campus.

Deppe, H.U., Gerhardt, U. and Novak, P. (eds) (1983) *Medizinische Soziologie Jahrbuch 3*. Frankfurt-am-Main, New York: Campus.

Derber, C. (ed.) (1982) *Professionals as Workers: Mental Labor in Advanced Capitalism*. Boston: G.K. Hall.

Derber, C. (1984) Physicians and their Sponsors: the New Medical Relations of Production. In McKinlay 1984: 217–54.

DeSantis, G. and Ferrera, M. (1983) *Composizione Partitica dei Comitati di Gestione delle USL*. Turin: Centro di Ricerca e Documentazione Luigi Einaudi.

Deutscher Partitätischer Wohlfahrtsverband (1985) *DPWV und Selbsthilfe-initiativen*. Wuppertal: DPWV.

DHSS (1979) *Patients First*. London: Department of Health and Social Security.

DHSS (1985) Management Budgeting in the NHS: Interim Report on Progress and Proposals for Further Development. London.

Döhler, Marian (1985) Entwicklungstendenzen und Probleme privater Gesundheitspolitik in den USA: das Beispiel der Health Care Coalitions. *Medizin-Mensch-Gesellschaft*, 10: 162–72.

Döhler, Marian (1986) Controlling the Doctor in Germany: on the Institutional Consolidation of Professional Power. Unpublished manuscript.

Donati, Pierpaolo P. (ed.) (1983) *La Sociologia Sanitaria*. Milan: Franco Angeli.

Douglas, M. and Wildavsky, A. (1982) *Risk and Culture*. Berkeley, Los Angeles: University of California Press.

Dudley, A. (1984) The DRG Tug-of-War. *Medicine and Computers*, September-October: 34–7.

Dumont, Jean-Pierre (1981) *La Sécurité Sociale: toujours en chantier*. Paris: Editions Ouvrières.

Dunham, Andrew B. and Marone, James A. (1984) The Politics of Innovation: the Evolution of DRG Rate Regulation in New Jersey. *DRG Evaluation IV-A*. Princeton, NJ: Health Research and Educational Trust of New Jersey.

Dyckman, Z.Y. (1978) A Study of Physicians' Fees. Washington, DC: Council on Wage and Price Stability.

Dyson, K. (1982) West Germany: the Search for a Rationalist Consensus. In Richardson 1982: 17–45.

Eckstein, H. (1979) On the 'Science' of the State. *Daedalus*, 108: 619–38.

Economist, The (1985) American Survey: Time for a Tourniquet on Medical Costs. 2 February: 19–21.

Edelman, Murray (1974) The Political Language of the Helping Professions. *Politics and Society*, 4: 295–320.

Ehrenreich, Barbara and Ehrenreich, John (1970) *The American Health Empire*. New York: Vintage Books.

Ehrenreich, John (1978) *The Cultural Crisis of Modern Medicine*. New York: Monthly Review Press.

Ehrmann, Henry W. (1983) *Politics in France* (4th edn). Boston, MA: Little, Brown.

Eimeren, W. van, Engelbrecht, R. and Flagle, C.D. (eds) (1984) *Third International Conference on System Science in Health Care*. Berlin, Heidelberg, New York, Tokyo: Springer.

Eisenstadt, S.M. and Rokkan, S. (1973) *Building States and Nations*. Beverly Hills, CA: Sage.

Elling, R.H. (1980) *Cross-National Study of Health Systems, Political Economies and Health Care*. New Brunswick, NJ: Transaction Books.

Elston, M.A. (1977) Medical Autonomy: Challenges and Responses. In Barnard and Lee 1977: 26–51.

Ensign, J. (1978) Third-Party Review Programs from the Blue Cross Vantage Point. *Journal of the American Medical Association*, 196: 188–91.

Enthoven, Alan (1978) Consumer Choice Health Plan. *New England Journal of Medicine*, 298: 650–8, 709–20.

Feder, Judith (1977) *Medicare: The Politics of Federal Health Insurance*. Lexington, MA: Lexington Books.

Feingold, Eugene (1977) Who Controls the Medical Care System? In Levin 1977: 193–9.

Feldstein, M.S. (1967) *Economic Analysis for Health Service Efficiency*. Amsterdam: North-Holland.

Ferber, C. von (1978) Soziale Selbstverwaltung. In Bogs and von Ferber 1978: 99–199.

Ferber, C. von (1985) Soziale Krankenversicherung im Wandel: Weiterentwicklung oder Strukturreform? *WSI Mitteilungen*, 10: 584–94.

Ferrera, Maurizio (1984) *Il Welfare State in Italia*. Bologna: Il Mulino.

Ferrera, Maurizio (1985) Verso un Servizio Sanitario Selettivo? *Stato e Mercato*, 14: 293–303.

Ferrera, Maurizio (1986) Italy. In Flora 1986: 385–499.

Ferrera, Maurizio and Zincone, G. (eds) (1986) *La Salute che noi Pensiamo: Domanda Sanitaria e Politiche Pubbliche in Italia*. Bologna: Il Mulino.

Festen, H. (1974) Honderdvijfentwintig jaar geneeskunst en Maatschappij. *Medisch Contact*, 29: 1305–20.

Field, Mark G. (1980) The Health System and the Polity: a Contemporary American Dialectic. *Social Science and Medicine*, 14A: 397–413.

Financial Survey (1987) *Financieel Overzicht Gezondheidszorg en Maatschappelijk Welzijn 1988* (Financial Survey of Health Care). Tweede Kamer, zitting 1987–8, 20209, nos. 1–2.

Flora, Peter (ed.) (1986) *Growth to Limits*: the Western European Welfare States since World War II. Berlin, New York: De Gruyter.

Francesconi, D. (1978) *Lavoratori e Organizzazione Sanitaria*. Bari: De Donato.

Freddi, Giorgio (1982) Historical Constraints on Administrative Performance: the Age Factor and the French, Italian and German Bureaucracies. *Studies in Public Organization*. Berkeley: Institute of Governmental Studies, University of California.

Freddi, Giorgio (ed.) (1984a) *Rapporto Perkoff: Salute e Organizzazione nel Servizio Sanitario Nazionale*. Bologna: Il Mulino.

Freddi, Giorgio (1984b) Conclusioni: il Servizio Sanitario come Sistema Politico-Organizzativo. In Freddi 1984a: 213–91.

Freddi, Giorgio (1986) Bureaucratic Rationalities and the Prospect for Party Government. In Castles and Wildemann 1986: 143–77.

Freidson, Eliot (ed.) (1963) *The Hospital in Modern Society*. New York: Free Press.

Freidson, Eliot (1970) *The Profession of Medicine: a Study of the Sociology of Applied Knowledge*. New York: Dodd, Mead.

Freidson, Eliot (1973) *Professional Dominance: the Social Structure of Medical Care*. Chicago: Aldine.

Freidson, Eliot (1975) *Doctoring Together*. New York: Elsevier.

Friedman, Milton (1962) *Capitalism and Freedom*. Chicago: University of Chicago Press.

Friedrich, Carl J. (1963) *Man and his Government: an Empirical Theory of Politics*. New York: McGraw-Hill.

Friend, J. and Noad, A. (1977) Inter-organizational Linkage: toward a Useful Theory. *Linkage*, 2: 18–20.

Fuchs, Victor R. (1974) *Who Shall Live? Health, Economics, and Social Choice*. New York: Basic Books.

Fuchs, Victor R. (1979) Economics, Health, and Post-Industrial Society. *Health and Society/Milbank Memorial Fund Quarterly*, 57: 153–82.

Fuchs, Victor R. (1982) The Battle for Control of Health Care. *Health Affairs*, 1(3): 5–13.

Gerstl, J. and Jacobs, G. (1975) *Professions for the People: the Politics of Skill*. New York: Schenkman.

Ginsburg, N. (1979) *Class, Capital and Social Policy*. London: Macmillan.

Glaser, William A. (1970) *Paying the Doctor*. Baltimore, MD: Johns Hopkins University Press.

Glaser, William A. (1978) *Health Insurance Bargaining: Foreign Lessons for Americans*. New York: Gardner Press.

Glaser, W.A. (1983) Lessons from Germany. *Journal of Health Politics, Policy and Law*, 8: 352–64.

Godt, P.J. (1985) Doctors and Deficits: Regulating the Medical Profession in France. *Public Administration*, 63: 151–69.

Goodman, J.C. (1980a) *National Health Care in Great Britain: Lessons for the USA*. Dallas, TX: Fisher Institute.

Goodman, J.C. (1980b) *The Regulation of Medical Care: Is the Price Too High?* San Francisco: Cato Institute.

Goran, M. (1979) Evolution of the PSRO Hospital Review System. *Medical Care*, Supplement 17.

Gray, Bradford (ed.) (1983) *New Health Care for Profit*. Washington, DC: National Academy Press.

Groth, Alexander J. and Wade, Larry L. (eds) (1985) *Public Policy across Nations: Social Welfare in Industrial Settings*. Greenwich, CT: JAI Press.

Hage, Jerry (1980) *Theories of Organizations: Form, Process and Transformation*. New York: Wiley.

Hage, Jerry and Hollingsworth, J.R. (1977) The First Steps toward the Integration of Social Theory and Social Policy. *Annals of the American Academy of Political and Social Science*, 434: 1–23.

Ham, C. (1985) *Health Policy in Britain* (2nd edn). London: Macmillan.

Hamm, W. (1980) *Irrwege der Gesundheitspolitik.* Tübingen: Mohr (Paul Seibeck).

Hammerström, A. and Janlert, U. (1983) Schweden. In Deppe 1983: 243–69.

Hanf, Kenneth and Scharpf, Fritz W. (eds) (1978) *Interorganizational Policy Making: Limits to Coordination and Central Control.* London: Sage.

Harrison, S., Pohlman, C. and Mercer, G. (1984) Concepts of Clinical Freedom amongst English Physicians. Paper presented at the European Association of Programmes in Health Services Studies, King Edward's Hospital Fund for London, 8 June.

Hatzfeld, Henri (1971) *Du paupérisme à la Sécurité Sociale 1850–1940.* Paris: Colin.

Haug, Marie and Lavin, Bebe (1983) *Consumerism in Medicine: Challenging Physician Authority.* Beverly Hills, CA: Sage.

Haywood, S. and Alaszewski, A. (1980) *Crisis in the Health Service.* London: Croom Helm.

Hegner, F. (1983) Sozialstationen: eine neue Organisationsform ambulanter Dienste im Wohnumfeld. In Deppe et al. 1983: 54–82.

Hegner, F. (1985a) Kommunale Initiativen zur Verwirklichung einer neuen Form der Vollbeschäftigung. In Krüger and Pankoke 1985: 241–66.

Hegner, F. (1985b) Arbeit im sozialen Bereich: Eigenhilfe, Ehrenamt, Berufsarbeit und Selbstorganisation. In Deutscher Partitätischer Wohlfahrtsverband 1985: 7–31.

Heidenheimer, Arnold J. (1973) The Politics of Public Education, Health and Welfare in the USA and Western Europe: How Growth and Reform Potential have Differed. *British Journal of Political Science*, 3: 315–41.

Heidenheimer, Arnold J. (1980) Conflict and Compromise between Professional and Bureaucratic Health Interests 1947–1972. In Heidenheimer and Elvander 1980: 119–42.

Heidenheimer, Arnold J. and Elvander, Nils (eds) (1980) *The Shaping of the Swedish Health System.* London: Croom Helm.

Herzlich, C. (1982) The Evolution of Relations between French Physicians and the State from 1880 to 1980. *Sociology of Health and Illness*, 4: 241–53.

Hessler, R.M. and Twaddle, A.C. (1982) Sweden's Crisis in Medical Care: Political and Legal Changes. *Journal of Health Politics, Policy and Law*, 7: 440–59.

Hessler, R.M. and Twaddle, A.C. (1986) Power and Change: Primary Health Care at the Crossroads in Sweden. *Human Organization*, 45: 134–47.

Hirschman, Albert O. (1970) *Exit, Voice, and Loyalty: Responses to Decline in Firms, Organizations, and States.* Cambridge, MA: Harvard University Press.

Hofland, J. and Wilms, P.J.M. (1984) *Onder Behandeling.* Deventer: Kluwer.

Höflich, J.R. (1984) *Kommunikation im Krankenhaus.* Augsburg: Maro.

Hogarth, J. (1963) *The Payment of General Practitioners.* New York: Pergamon.

Hollingsworth, J.R. (1982) The Political Structural Basis for Economic Performance. *Annals of the American Academy of Political and Social Science*, 459: 20–45.

Hollingsworth, J.R. (1986) *The Political Economy of Medicine: Great Britain and the US.* Baltimore, MD: Johns Hopkins University Press.

Hollingsworth, J.R. and Hanneman, R. (1983) *Centralization and Power in Social Delivery Systems: the Cases of England, Wales, and the United States,* Boston, MA: Kluwer-Nijhoff.

Hollingsworth, J.R., Hage, J. and Hanneman, R. (1978) The Impact of the Organization of Health Delivery Systems on Health Efficiency: a Comparative Analysis of the United States, France, and Great Britain. Paper presented at the American Sociological Association, San Francisco.

Honigh, M. (1985) *Doeltreffend Beleid: een Empirische Vergelijking van Beleids-sectoren.* Assen, Maastricht: Van Gorcum.

Hunt, K. (1983) DRG – What it is, How it Works, and Why it will Hurt. *Medical Economics,* 5 September: 264–5.

Illich, I. (1977) *Limits to Medicine.* Harmondsworth: Pelican.

Jaques, Eliot (ed.) (1978) *Health Services: their Nature and Organisation and Role of Patients, Doctors, Nurses, and the Complementary Professions.* London: Heinemann.

Jamous, Haroun (1969) *Sociologie de la décision: la réforme des études médicales et des structures hospitalières.* Paris: Editions du Centre National de la Recherche.

Johnson, N. (1979) Quangos and the Structure of British Government. *Public Administration,* 57: 379–95.

Johnson, T.J. (1972) *Professions and Power.* London: Macmillan.

Jordan, G. and Richardson, J. (1982) The British Policy Style or the Logic of Negotiation. In Richardson 1982: 80–109.

Juffermans, P. (1982) *Staat en Gezondheidszorg in Nederland.* Nijmegen: SUN.

Katz, R.S. (ed.) (1987) *Party Governments: European and American Experiences.* Berlin, New York: de Gruyter.

Kelman, S. (1981) *Regulating America, Regulating Sweden: a Comparative Study of Occupational Safety and Health Policy.* Cambridge, MA: MIT Press.

Kervasdoué, Jean de and Rodwin, Victor (1981) La Politique de santé et le rôle de l'état: 1945–1980. In Kervasdoué et al. 1981: 39–57.

Kervasdoué, Jean de, Rodwin, Victor G. and Kimberley, John R. (eds) (1981) *La Santé rationnée?* Paris: Economica.

Kessel, R.A. (1959) Price Discrimination in Medicine. *Journal of Law and Economics,* 1: 20–51.

Kessel, R.A. (1970) The AMA and the Supply of Physicians. *Law and Contemporary Problems,* 35: 267–83.

Keupp, Heinrich and Rerrisch, Dodo (eds) (1982) *Psychosoziale Praxis: Gemeinde-psychologische Perspektiven.* Munich: Urban und Schwarzenberg.

Kickbusch, I. and Trojan, A. (eds) (1981) *Gemeinsam sind wir Stärker: Selbsthilfe-gruppen und Gesundheit.* Frankfurt-am-Main: Fischer Alternative.

Klein, Rudolf (1977) The Corporate State, Health Service, and the Professions. *New University Quarterly,* 31: 161–80.

Klein, Rudolf (1980) The Welfare State: a Self-Inflicted Crisis? *Political Quarterly,* 51: 24–34.

Klein, Rudolf (1983a) *The Politics of the National Health Service.* London: Longman.

Klein, Rudolf (1983b) The NHS and the Theatre of Inadequacy. *University Quarterly,* 37: 201–15.

Koenen, E. and Riedmüller, B. (1982) Sozialpolitik und psychosoziale Versorgung. In Keupp and Rerrisch 1982: 97–106.

Kornhauser, W. (1962) *Scientists in Industry.* Berkeley: University of California Press.

Krause, E. (1977) *Power and Illness: the Political Sociology of Health and Medical Care.* New York: Elsevier.

Krebs, K.H. and John, J. (1985) Economic Appraisal of Health Technology: Country Statement: Federal Republic of Germany. Paper prepared for an EC Workshop on the Methodology of Economic Appraisal of Health Technology, Birmingham, England.

Krizay, John and Wilson, Andrew (1974) *The Patient as Consumer*. Lexington, MA: Lexington Books.

Krüger, J. and Pankoke, E. (eds) (1985) *Kommunale Sozialpolitik*. Munich: Oldenbourg.

Kuty, O. (1973) Le Pouvoir du malade: analyse sociologique des unités de rein artificiel. Doctoral thesis, Université Descartes, Paris.

Labisch, A. (1985) Gesundheitssicherung in der Gemeinde – Tradition, Stand, Aufgaben für die Zukunft. Paper for a meeting of Deutschen Zentrale für Volksgesundheitspflege e.V., 27 February, Frankfurt-am-Main.

Landau, M. (1969) Redundancy, Rationality and the Problem of Duplication and Overlap. *Public Administration Review*, 29: 346–58.

Landau, M. (1973) On the Concept of a Self-Correcting Organization. *Public Administration Review*, 33: 533–44.

Landau, M. (1985) On Multi-Organizational Systems in Public Administration. *Rivista Trimestrale de Scienza dell'Amministrazione*, 32: 3–20.

Landstingsförbundet (1973–83) *Landstingsanställd personal*. Stockholm: Landstingsförbundet.

Larkin, G. (1983) *Occupational Monopoly and Modern Medicine*. London: Tavistock.

Law, Sylvia A. (1974) *Blue Cross: What Went Wrong?* New Haven, CT: Yale University Press.

Lebish, D.J. (1982) PSROs and Utilization Review: Life, Death, and Rebirth. In Cleverly 1982: 986–98.

LeGrand, J. (1978) The Distribution of Public Expenditure: the Case of Health Care. *Economica*, 45: 125–48.

Lehmbruch, G. and Schmitter, Philippe C. (eds) (1982) *Patterns of Corporatist Policy-Making*. Beverly Hills, CA: Sage.

Lehner, F. and Widmaier, V. (1983) Market Failure and Growth of Government: a Sociological Explanation. In Taylor 1983: 118–37.

Leibfried, S. and Tennstedt, F. (eds) (1985) *Politik der Armut und die Spaltung des Sozialstaats*. Frankfurt-am-Main: Suhrkamp.

Leichter, Howard M. (1979) *A Comparative Approach to Policy Analysis: Health Care Policy in Four Nations*. New York: Cambridge University Press.

Levin, Arthur (ed.) (1977) *Health Services: the Local Perspective*. New York: Academy of Political Science.

Levin, Arthur (ed.) (1980) *Regulating Health Care: the Struggle for Control*. New York: Academy of Political Science.

Levitt, Ruth (1977) *The Reorganized National Health Service* (2nd edn). London: Croom Helm.

Levy, S. and Hesse, D.D. (1985) Bottom-Line Health Care? *New England Journal of Medicine*, 312: 963–70.

Lijphart, A. (1968) *The Politics of Accommodation*. Berkeley: University of California Press.

Long, A.F. and Harrison, S. (1985) *Health Services Performance*. London: Croom Helm.

Lowi, Theodore J. (1974) Four Systems of Policy, Politics and Choice. *Public Administration Review*, 4: 298–310.

Lowi, Theodore J. (1979) *The End of Liberalism: the Second Republic of the United States*. New York: W.W. Norton.

Luft, Harold D. (1983) Economic Incentives and Clinical Decisions. In Gray 1983: 103–23.

McKinlay, J.B. (ed.) (1984) *Issues in the Political Economy of Health Care*. New York, London: Tavistock.

McKnight, Jack (1975) *The Medicalization of Politics*. Zürich: Gottlieb Duttweiler Institut.

McLachlan, Gordon and Maynard, Alan (eds) (1982) *The Public/Private Mix for Health*. London: Nuffield Provincial Hospitals Trust.

Mackensen, R. and Sagebeil, F. (eds) (1979) *Soziologische Analysen*. Berlin: TU Berlin.

Marcson, S. (1960) *The Scientist in American Industry*. Princeton: Industrial Relations Section, Princeton University.

Marmor, Theodore R. (1973) *The Politics of Medicare*. Chicago: Aldine and London: Routledge & Kegan Paul.

Marmor, Theodore R. (1976) Congress Adopts Medicare. In Anderson 1976: 119–43.

Marmor, Theodore R. (1983) *Political Analysis and American Medical Care*. Cambridge: Cambridge University Press.

Marmor, Theodore R. and Christenson, Jon (1982) *The Politics of Health Care*. Beverly Hills, CA: Sage.

Marmor, Theodore R. and Thomas, D. (1972) Doctors, Politics and Pay Disputes: 'Pressure Group Politics' Revisited. *British Journal of Political Science*, 2: 422–42.

Marone, James and Dunham, Andrew (1983) The Emerging Autonomy of the State: Health Politics and the Hospital Industry. Paper presented at the Annual Meeting of the American Political Science Association, Chicago, 1–4 September.

Marone, James and Dunham, Andrew (1984) The Waning of Professional Dominance: DRGs and the Hospitals. *Health Affairs*, 3: 73–86.

Martinelli, A. (1983) Salute e Sistemi Sanitari Occidentale. In Donati 1983: 121–40.

Marx, Karl and Engels, Friedrich (1969) Werke. Berlin: Dietz.

May, J. J. and Wasserman, J. (1985). Selected Results from an Evaluation of the New Jersey Diagnosis-Related Research Group System. *Health Services Research*, 19: 547–59.

Maynard, Alan (1984) The Implications of Economic Constraints on Clinical Autonomy. Paper presented at the Conference on Clinical Autonomy, European Association of Programmes in Health Service Studies, London, King's Fund Centre.

Mayntz, R, Klitzach, W. and Oberländer, E. (1982) *Analyse von Planungs- und Steuerungsfunktionen der gesetzlichen Krankenversicherung in Versorgungsschwerpunkten des Gesundheitswesens*. Gesundheitsforschung, 69. Bonn: Bundesminister für Arbeit und Sozialordnung.

Mechanic, David (1976) *The Growth of Bureaucratic Medicine*. New York: Wiley.

Memorandum (1974) *Structuurnota Gezondheidszorg* (Memorandum on the Structure of the Health Services). Tweede Kamer, zitting 1973–4, 13012, nos. 1–2.

Mény, Yves (1985) La Légitimation des groupes d'intérêt par l'administration française. *Proceedings of the XIIIth World Congress of the International Political Science Association*, Paris.

Merschbrock-Bäuerle, A., Redler-Hasford, E. and van Eimeren, W. (1985) Gesundheitspolitik für alte Menschen in der Bundesrepublik Deutschland. MEDIS, Munich, unpublished manuscript.

Meynaud, Jean (1962) Les Groupes de pression sous la Vème République. *Revue Française de Science Politique*, 12: 672–97.

Mignot, Gabriel and d'Orsay, P. (1968) *La Machine administrative*. Paris: Seuil.

Miller, R.D. (1983) *Problems in Hospital Law*. Rockville, MD: Aspen Systems.

Millerson, G. (1964) Dilemmas of Professionalism. *New Society*, 4 June.

Mills, C. Wright (1956) *The Power Elite.* New York: Oxford University Press.
Moore, Wilbert E. (1970) *The Professions: Roles and Rules.* New York: Russell Sage Foundation.
Mosher, Frederick (1978) Professions in Public Service. *Public Administration Review,* 38: 144–50.
Müller, J. and Wasem, J. (1984) Missing Links zwischen Ambulanter und Stationärer Versorgung im Ärtzlichen und Pflegerischen Bereich. *Archiv für Wissenschaft und Praxis,* Special isue for 2/1984.
Müller, U. (1979) Verrechtlichung medizinischen Handelns. Deprofessionalisierungsprozesse im Berufsfeld Medizin. In Mackensen and Sagebeil 1979: 193–9.
Muntendam, P. (1983) Gezondheidszorg in Ontwikkeling. In Schrijvers and Boot 1983: 21–53.
Naschold, Frieder (1976) Strukturelle Bestimmungsfaktoren für die Kostenentwicklung im Gesundheitswesen. *Das Argument,* 12: 196–206.
Neubauer, G. (1985) Wahlen als Steuerungs- und Kontrollinstrument der Gemeinsamen Selbstverwaltung. Paper presented at the Jahrestagung Ökonomie des Gesundheitswesens, Verein für Socialpolitik, Saarbrücken.
Neubauer, G. and Rebscher, H. (1984) *Gemeinsame Selbstverwaltung.* Spardorf: René F. Wilfer.
Newhouse, J.P. et al. (1982) *Some Interim Results from a Controlled Trial of Cost Sharing in Health Insurance.* Santa Monica, CA: Rand.
NHS Management Inquiry (1983) *Report.* London: DHSS.
Nobrega, F.T. and Krishnan, I. (1983) The Impact of Regulation and Competition on the Quality of Health Care: a Physician's Perspective. *Mayo Clinic Proceedings,* 58: 834–7.
Nord, D. (1982) *Die soziale Steuerung der Arzneimittelversorgung.* Stuttgart: F. Enke.
Oates, W.E. (1972) *Fiscal Federalism.* New York: Harcourt Brace Jovanovich.
Oetzel, E.-A. (1981) Einigungsverhandlungen aus der Sicht der Landesbehörden. *Krankenhaus-Umschau,* 140–7.
Office of Health Economics (1981) *Compendium of Health Statistics.* 3rd edn. London.
Olson, Mancur (1965) *The Logic of Collective Action.* Cambridge, MA: Harvard University Press.
Ostrom, Vincent (1983) Nonhierarchical Approaches to the Organization of Public Activity. *Annals of the American Academy of Political and Social Science,* 466: 135–47.
Pasquino, G.F. (1987) Party Government in Italy: Achievements and Prospects. In Katz 1987: 202–41.
Pear, Robert (1985) Companies Tackle Health Costs. *The New York Times,* 3 March: 1.
Perkoff, G. (1979) *Changing Health Care: Perspectives from a New Medical Care Setting.* Ann Arbor: University of Michigan Press.
Perkoff, G. (1984) Efficienza e Efficacia del Servizio Sanitario: Condizioni Professionali e Organizzativo-Istituzionali. In Freddi 1984a: 21–117.
Perrow, C. (1961) Organisational Prestige: Some Functions and Dysfunctions. *American Journal of Sociology,* 66: 335–41.
Perrow, C. (1963) Goals and Power Structure: a Historical Case Study. In Freidson 1963: 112–46.
Peters, T.J. and Waterman, R.H. (1983) *In Search of Excellence.* New York: Harper & Row.

Piperno, A. (1983) Medici e Stato in Italia. In Donati 1983: 141–63.

Piperno, A. (1984). La Politica Sanitaria. In Ascoli 1984: 153–84.

Piperno, A. (ed.) (1986) *La Politica Sanitaria in Italia*. Milan: Angeli.

Pohlman, C. (1985) Clinical Autonomy and Health Service Management: Medical Perspectives on Management in the British National Health Service. Paper towards MHA degree, University of Wisconsin–Madison.

Polsby, Nelson (1975) Legislatures. In Polsby and Greenstein 1975: 257–319.

Polsby, Nelson and Greenstein, Fred I. (eds) (1975) *Handbook of Political Science*. Boston: Addison-Wesley.

Potthoff, P. and Leidl, R. (1986) Kassenärztliche Einweisungen und Entwicklungen im Krankenhaussektor. In Schwefel et al. 1986a: 215–31.

Raffel, Marshall W. (1980) *The US Health System: Origins and Functions*. New York: Wiley.

Rathwell, T. and Barnard, K. (1985) Health Services Performance in Britain. In Long and Harrison 1985: 126–62.

Rauskolb, Ch. (1976) *Lobby in Weiß: Struktur und Politik der Ärzteverbände*. Frankfurt-am-Main: Europäische Verlagsanstalt.

Reimann, H. and Reimann, H. (eds) (1976) *Medizinische Versorgung*. Munich: Goldmann.

Richardson, Jeremy (ed.) (1982) *Policy Styles in Western Europe*. London: Allen & Unwin.

Riedmüller, B. (1980) Der gemeindepsychiatrische Dienst im Widerspruch zwischen professionellen und nicht-professionellen Hilfen. *Leviathan*, 4: 518–37.

Robinson, M. (1982) New Regs Spur Monitoring of MDs. *Modern Health Care*, December: 20.

Robson, J. (1973) The NHS Company Inc? The Social Consequences of the Professional Dominance in the National Health Service. *International Journal of Health Services*, 3: 413–26.

Rodwin, Victor G. (1981) The Marriage of National Health Insurance and 'la Médecine Libérale' in France: a Costly Union. *Health and Society/Milbank Memorial Fund Quarterly*, 59: 16–43.

Rodwin, Victor G. (1982) Management without Objectives: the French Health Policy Gamble. In McLachlan and Maynard 1982: 287–325.

Rohde, J.J. (1967) *Zur Soziologie des Krankenhauses*. Stuttgart: Kohlhammer.

Rose, Richard (1984a) *Understanding Big Government*. London: Sage.

Rose, Richard (1984b) *Comparative Policy Analysis: the Programme Approach*. Studies in Public Policy 138, Centre for the Study of Public Policy, University of Strathclyde.

Rothstein, William (1972) *American Physicians in the 19th Century: from Sects to Science*. Baltimore, MD: Johns Hopkins University Press.

Royal Commission (1979) *Report of the Royal Commission on the National Health Service*. Cmnd 7615. London: HMSO.

Rueschemeyer, Dietrich (1964) Doctors and Lawyers: a Comment on the Theory of the Professions. *Canadian Review of Sociology and Anthropology*, 1: 17–30.

Rutten, F. and van der Werff, A. (1982) Health Policy in the Netherlands: at the Crossroads. In McLachlan and Maynard 1982: 167–207.

Sacconi, L. (ed.) (1986) *La Decisione: Razionalità Collectiva e Strategia nell' Amministrazione e nelle Organizzazioni*. Milan: Franco Angeli.

Saltman, R.B. (1983) Resource-Related Decisions inside Two Swedish Central County Hospitals: Some Initial Impressions. Unpublished manuscript, Göteborg.

Saltman, R.B. and Young, D. (1981) The Hospital Power Equilibrium: an

Alternative View of the Cost Containment Dilemma. *Journal of Health Politics, Policy and Law*, 6: 392–6.

Salvati, M. (1981) *Alle Origini dell'Inflazione Italiana*. Bologna: Il Mulino.

Sandier, S. and Stephan, J.-C. (1983) Frankreich. In Deppe 1983: 65–103.

Satzinger, W. (1986a) Der Bayern-Vertrag: Ziele, Hintergrund, Programm. In Schwefel et al. 1986a: 1–23.

Satzinger, W. (1986b) Der Bayern-Vertrag in der gesundheitspolitischen Entwicklung: Trendmacher, Trendfolger, Trendopponent? In Schwefel et al. 1986a: 843–943.

Satzinger, W., Leidl, R. and Lindenmüller, H. (1984) The Anti-Hospital Bias in West German Hospital Policy: a Reaction to Economic Trend or a New Trend in Medical Care? In Eimeren et al. 1984: 651–3.

Scase, R. (1977) *Social Democracy in Capitalist Society*. London: Croom Helm.

Scharpf, F.W. (1985) *The Joint Decision Trap: Lessons from German Federalism and European Integration*. Wissenschaftszentrum, Berlin, report IIM/LMP 85–1.

Scharpf, F.W., Reissert, B. and Schnabel, F. (1978) Policy Effectiveness and Conflict Avoidance in Intergovernmental Policy Formation. In Hanf and Scharpf 1978: 57–112.

Schattschneider, E.E. (1960) *The Semi-Sovereign People*. New York: Holt Rinehart.

Schmitter, Philippe and Lehmbruch, Gerhard (eds) (1979) *Trends toward Corporatist Intermediation*. Beverly Hills, CA: Sage.

Schnabel, F. (1980) Politischer und Administrativer Vollzug des Krankenhaus-finanzierungsgesetzes. Dissertation, University of Konstanz.

Schön, A., Kopetzky, D., Janzer, H. and Schwab, G. (1978). Analyse und Bewertung der Krankenhausbedarfspläne der deutschen Bundesländer. *Das Krankenhaus*, 159–66, 224–35.

Schrijvers, G. and Boot, J.M. (eds) (1983) *Een Halve Eeuw Gezondheidszorg*. Lochem: De Tijdstroom.

Schroeder, S.A. (1980) Variation in Physician Practice Patterns: a Review of Medical Cost Implications. In Carels et al. 1980: 23–50.

Schulenburg, J.M. Graf der (1983) Report from Germany: Current Conditions and Controversies in the Health Care System. *Journal of Health Politics, Policy and Law*, 8: 320–51.

Schulenburg, J.M. Graf der (1984) *Selbstregulierung durch Berufsverbände: eine Studie am Beispiel des Gesundheitswesens*. Wissenschaftszentrum, Berlin.

Schülke, H. (1977) Die Verhandlungen zwischen Kassernärztlichen Vereinigungen und Krankenkassen. MA thesis, University of Konstanz.

Schulz, R.I. and Scheckler, W.E. (1988) Physician Concerns and Experience with the Incorporation of Health Maintenance Organizations into Private Practice. Mimeo, Department of Preventive Medicine, University of Wisconsin–Madison.

Schulz, R.I., Harrison, S., Pohlman, C., Scheckler, W.E. and Mercer, G. (1985) Physician Autonomy: Comparisons between a Competitive and a Nationalised Health System. Paper for Joint Sessions of Workshops, European Consortium for Political Research, Barcelona, 26 March.

Schwefel, D. (1985) Effektivitäten von Steuerungspolitiken im Gesundheitswesen. Paper delivered at the Jahrestagung Ökonomie des Gesundheitswesens, Verein für Sozialpolitik, Saarbrücken, 16–18 September.

Schwefel, D., van Eimeren, W. and Satzinger, W. (1986a) *Der Bayern-Vertrag: Evaluation einer Kostendämpfungspolitik im Gesundheitswesen*. Berlin: Springer.

Schwefel, D., van Eimeren, W., Satzinger, W., Potthoff, P., John, J., Merschbrock-Bäuerle, A. and Zwerenz, K. (1986b) Auswirkungen und Wirksamkeit des Bayern-Vertrags: Zusammenfassung von Evaluationsergebnissen. In Schwefel et al. 1986a: 945–85.

Serner, Uncas (1980) Swedish Health Legislation: Milestones in Reorganization. In Heidenheimer and Elvander 1980: 99–117.

Shenkin, B.N. (1973) Politics and Medical Care in Sweden: the Seven Crowns Reform. *New England Journal of Medicine*, 288: 555–9.

Shryock, Richard (1967) *Medical Licensing in America, 1650–1965*. Baltimore, MD: Johns Hopkins University Press.

Siebig, J. (1981) Funktionsprobleme einer kooperativen Gesundheitspolitik: der Fall 'Konzertierte Aktion'. *Krankenhaus-Umschau*, 2: 79–84.

Siegrist, J. (1978) *Arbeit und Interaktion im Krankenhaus*. Stuttgart: Enke.

Simborg, D.W. (1981) DRG-Creep: a New Hospital Acquired Disease. *New England Journal of Medicine*, 296: 1602–4.

Simon, H. (1947) *Administrative Behavior*. New York: Macmillan.

Simon, H. (1960) *The New Science of Management Decision*. New York: Harper.

Skidmore, Max J. (1970) *Medicare and the American Rhetoric of Reconciliation*. Alabama: University of Alabama Press.

SOU (1979: 78). *Mål och medel för hälso- och sjukvården*. Stockholm: Socialdepartmentet.

SOU (1981: 2). *Ohälsa och vårdutnyttjande*. Stockholm: Socialdepartmentet.

Speller, S.R. (1965) *Law Relating to Hospitals and Kindred Institutions*. London: H.K. Lewis.

Stacey, M. (ed.) (1976) *The Sociology of the National Health Service*. Keele: University Press.

Starr, Paul (1982) *The Social Transformation of American Medicine: the Rise of a Sovereign Profession and the Making of a Vast Industry*. New York: Basic Books.

Steudler, F. (1977) Médecine libérale et conventionnement. *Sociologie du Travail*, 17: 176–98.

Steudler, F. (1984) L'État et la santé. *Prospective et Santé*, 29: 11–26.

Stevens, Rosemary (1976) The Evolution of the Health-Care Systems in the United States and the United Kingdom: Similarities and Differences. In Fogarty International Center Proceedings, *Priorities for the Use of Resources in Medicine*. Bethesda, MD: US Department of Health, Education and Welfare.

Stone, Deborah A. (1980) *The Limits of Professional Power: National Health Insurance in the Federal Republic of Germany*. Chicago: University of Chicago Press.

Suleiman, Ezra N. (1974) *Politics, Power and Bureaucracy in France: the Administrative Elite*. Princeton, NJ: Princeton University Press.

Taylor, C.L. (ed.) (1983) *Why Governments Grow: Measuring Public Sector Size*. Beverly Hills, CA: Sage.

Tennstedt, F. (1977) *Soziale Selbstverwaltung*. Bonn: Ortskrankenkassen.

Thiemeyer, T. (1979) *Analyse und Neugestaltung der Pauschalen für Instandhaltung und Instandsetzung nach der Bundespflegesatzverordnung*. Gesundheitsforschung 11. Bonn: Bundesminister für Arbeit und Sozialordnung.

Thiemeyer, T. (1981) *Einordnung von Krankenhäusern in ein Abgestuftes Versorgungssystem*. Forschungsstätte für öffentliche und private Unternehmen e.V. Bochum: Ruhr Universität.

Thompson, Frank J. (1981) *Health Policy and the Bureaucracy: Policies and Implementation*. Boston: MIT Press.

Tiemann, S. (1983) *Ärztliche Freiberuflichkeit im Spannungsfeld sozialversicherungsrechtlicher Regelungen*. Informationsdienst no. 153. Köln: Gesellschaft für Versicherungswissenschaft und -gestaltung e.V.

Titmuss, Richard (1974) *Social Policy: an Introduction*. London: Allen & Unwin.

Tolliday, H. (1978) Clinical Autonomy. In Jaques 1978: 32–52.

Verandering verzekerd (1988) Tweede Kamer, vergaderjaar 1987–8, 19945, nos. 27–8.

Verdoorn, J.A. (1981) *Het Gezondheidswezen te Amsterdam in de 19e Eeuw.* Nijmegen: SUN.

Wallace, C. (1984) Government, PROs Racing to Implement Touch Review System. *Modern Health Care,* October: 44.

Waller, H. (1985) Integration sozialer und medizinischer Dienste: Beispiele Gemeindenaher Versorgung in der Bundesrepublik Deutschland. *WSI Mitteilungen,* 10: 500–606.

Watkin, B. (1979) *The NHS: the First Phase,* 1948–1974. London: Allen & Unwin.

Wennberg, Jack, Barnes, B. and Zubkoff, Michael (1982) Professional Uncertainty and the Problem of Supplier-Induced Demand. *Social Science and Medicine,* 16: 811–24.

Wennberg, Jack, McPherson, K. and Caper, P. (1984) Will Payments Based on Diagnosis Related Groups Control Hospital Costs? *New England Journal of Medicine,* 311: 295–300.

Wiesenthal, H. (1981) *Die konzertierte Aktion im Gesundheitswesen: ein Beispiel für Theorie und Politik des modernen Korporatismus.* Frankfurt-am-Main, New York: Campus.

Wildavsky, A. (1972) The Self-Evaluating Organization. *Public Administration Review,* 32: 509–20.

Wildavsky, A. (1986) Doing More and Using Less: Utilization of Research as a Result of a Regime. *Rivista Trimestriale di scienze dell'Amministrazione,* 3: 3–52.

Willcocks, A.J. (1967) *The Creation of the NHS.* London: Routledge & Kegan Paul.

Wilsford, David (1984) Exit and Voice: Strategies for Change in Bureaucratic-Legislative Policymaking. *Policy Studies Journal,* 12: 431–44.

Wilsford, David (1985) The Conjuncture of Ideas and Interests: a Note on Explanations of the French Revolution. *Comparative Political Studies,* 18: 357–72.

Wilsford, David (1988) Tactical Advantages versus Administrative Heterogeneity: the Strengths and the Weaknesses of the French State. *Comparative Political Studies,* 21(1): 126–68.

Wilson, Frank L. (1983) French Interest Group Politics: Pluralist or Neocorporatist? *American Political Science Review,* 77(4): 895–910.

WiPRO Reviewer (1984) *WiPRO Reviewer,* 1 (August): 6.

Wohl, S. (1984) *The Medical Industrial Complex.* New York: Harmony Books.

Wolff, L. de (1984) *De Prijs voor Gezondheid: het Centraal Orgaan Ziekenhuistarieven 1965–1982.* Baarn: Ambo.

WSI Mitteilungen (1985) Gesundheitspolitik in der Wende-Marktillusion oder Strukturreform? *WSI Mitteilungen: Zeitschrift des Wirtschafts- und Sozialwissenschaftlichen Instituts des Gewerkschaftsbundes.* Special issue.

Wuster, W. (1985) Die Selbstverwaltung der Gesetzlichen Krankenversicherung: Wandel, Macht und Ohnmacht. *WSI Mitteilungen,* 10: 614–21.

Wylie, Laurence (1957) *Village in the Vaucluse.* Cambridge, MA: Harvard University Press.

Zacher, H.F. (1985) Arzt und Sozialstaat. *Sozialer Fortschritt,* 10: 217–24.

Zimmer, C.L. (1985) Zur neuen Bundespflegesatzverordnung (BPflV). *Krankenhaus-Umschau,* 10: 759–65.

Zubkoff, Michael (ed.) (1976) *Health: a Victim or Cause of Inflation?* New York: Milbank Memorial Fund.

Index

Aaron, H.J. and Schwartz, W.B., 202
access to health care, 1, 9, 23, 26, 130, 211–12, 214–17, 224–5; Britain, 214, 224–5, 228; France, 190; Italy, 127–8; Sweden, 86, 192; US, 39–40, 46, 60, 69–70, 214, 224, 228
accountability, 28, 29–30, 31, 54, 129, 170
accreditation, 25, 107, 111, 203–4
administration: Britain, 187; as bureaucracy, 11, 26, 31–2, 112, 118; direct, 21; France, 16–17, 136; Germany, 14; and health service power, 2, 17, 60–1, 69, 78–81, 86, 118; Italy, 129; and physicians, 9, 32, 49–50, 56, 64–7, 213; Sweden, 78, 79, 80, 84, 90–1, 92–4, 97–8
admission, criteria for, 59
agent, physician as, 48, 65–6
Alford, R.R., 199, 200, 209
American Hospital Association, 51–2, 56, 61–2
American Medical Association, 21, 33–7, 52, 54–5, 60–5, 68, 71, 120, 141–2, 182–3
Anderson, O.W. and Shields, M., 53, 65
associations, medical: Britain, see British Medical Association; France, 142–7, see also Confédération des Syndicats Médicaux Français, Fédération des Médecins de France; Germany, 185; as interest groups, 5, 9, 14, 16–17, 114, 134, 137–9, 141–7, 149–55; Italy, 20, 123; Sweden, 18, 77, 193–4, see also Swedish Medical Association; US, 22, see also American Medical Association
autonomy: of central and local government, 81–3, 84, 88, 93, 213; hospitals, 162
autonomy, medical, 2–5
  clinical, 5, 6–8, 9, 17, 18, 20–2, 23, 25–6, 180, 195, 198–209; Britain, 189, 200–3, 206; France, 140; Germany, 186–7; Sweden, 17–18, 88–9, 90–4, 96–7; US, 30, 33–9, 46–50, 50–1, 56–7, 64, 66–9, 72, 183–4, 195, 203–5
  criteria, 5–9, 20, 29, 198, 199–200
  institutional environment, 3, 7–8, 10, 18–20, 23, 90–1; see also organization
  and political environment, 3, 10, 14–22, 23, 30–3, 74, 118; France, 138–9; Italy, 123, 126, 127; Netherlands, 112; Sweden, 81–3, 83–7, 91–4
  and welfare state, 178–97
  see also control, political; professionals, medical; and under individual countries

Barzach, M., 141
Bavarian Contract, 164, 177
Beer, S.H., 61–2
Bennett, W., 54–5, 56
Berlinguer, E., 18, 121
Blue Cross (US), 37–8, 51–2, 54
Britain: medical autonomy, 17, 128, 187–9,

220; political culture, 13, 14, 26–7, 118–19, 127; see also national health service
British Medical Association (BMA), 119, 188
budget financing, 94, 109, 161, 201
budgeting, management, 206
bureaucracy, see administration

cabinets, France, 135–6
Caisse Nationale d'Assurance Maladie des Travailleurs Salariés (CNAM), 189–91
capital formation: Germany, 162; Netherlands, 102, 105; Sweden, 84–5; US, 41, 43
Carder, M. and Klingeberg, B., 194
casse mutue, Italy, 116, 121–4, 126
Central Health Council, Netherlands, 102, 113–14
Central Organization for Health Tariffs, Netherlands, 104, 108–10, 113–14
Central Organization for Hospital Tariffs (COZ), Netherlands, 15, 103, 113–14
centralization, 26, 73, 74, 215–17; Britain, 119, 221–3, 226–7; France, 16, 142, 189–90; Germany, 167–70; and innovation, 17, 27, 215–16, 222, 226–7; Italy, 127; Netherlands, 113; Sweden, 83, 86–7, 95–6; US, 61, 64, 69, 221
Christian Democratic Party (DC), Italy, 121–5, 126
CNEL, Italy, 122, 123, 125
collectivism, hierarchical, 10, 11, 13, 14–16, 21, 194
Communist Party (PCI), Italy, 13, 18–19, 121–2, 125–6
community health, 8, 94, 127–8
competition, regulation by, 47, 61
Confédération des Syndicats Médicaux Français (CSMF), 139, 142–4, 146–7, 150–1, 153, 190–1
consensus model, 5, 9
consultation, state/physicians, 16–17, 109, 147–9, 152, 157
consumer interests, 2, 33, 70, 109–11, 129, 200, 211, 213–14, 218–22, 224–5; see also doctor–patient relationship; provider–consumer relationship
control, political: Britain, 73, 213, 223; France, 120, 147–52, 156; Germany, 157–73, 176, 180; Italy, 128–9; Netherlands, 99–100, 102, 104–11, 112–14; Sweden, 83–5, 87, 90–1, 94, 97–8, 194; US, 30–3, 39, 44, 46–67, 69–72, 182, 213; and welfare state, 178–80; see also autonomy, medical; and under individual countries
cooperation/contest, state vs physicians, 147, 150–1, 152, 153–4
corporatism, 21; consociational, 15, 99, 114; Germany, 14–15, 157–9, 161, 164, 172, 176,

186, 196; Netherlands, 15, 99, 114; Sweden, 192

Coser, R.L., 7

cost containment, 1, 23, 215–16; Britain, 17, 201, 205–6, 225; France, 132, 190–2; Germany, 162–3, 167, 171, 186, 196–7; Netherlands, 103–4, 108–10, 112–13; and physician power, 49–50, 178–9; US, 21–2, 39–41, 43–7, 51–6, 58, 60–2, 66–70, 182–4, 204–5, 207–8; and welfare state, 178–9, 196–7

costs, expansion: Britain, 225; France, 131–3, 196; Germany, 14, 163–4; Italy, 123–4; Netherlands, 111–12; and physicians' decisions, 178–9, 189; Sweden, 75, 76, 194; US, 39–41, 44, 46–7, 58, 182–3, 204, 207–8, 223

Council of Hospital Facilities, Netherlands, 104, 105–7, 111–12, 113, 115

Cross Societies, Netherlands, 100–1, 103–4

Crozier, M., 26, 49

decentralization: France, 133, 140; Germany, 158, 160, 168, 176–7; Italy, 19, 125, 127, 128–9; Netherlands, 107, 111–12; Sweden, 18, 74, 84, 86–8, 89, 91–4, 95–8, 119–20; US, 37, 182, 205, 215–16, 221–2

decision-making, *see* planning

Delogu, S., 121

demand: France, 130–1, 133; Italy, 127; US, 35, 46–7

diagnostic-related groups (DRGs), 21, 45–6, 58–63, 66–9, 72, 184, 207

direct action, France, 149–52, 155; *see also* strikes

doctor–patient relationship, 5, 31, 37, 41, 48, 55, 195

doctors, autonomy of, *see* autonomy, medical

Dole, Robert, 61

Douglas, M. and Wildavsky, A., 10. 12

efficiency, economic, 41, 44, 57, 185–6, 196

Ehrmann, H.W., 147

employment in health sector, Sweden, 75, 80, 81, 82

equality: legal, 10–11; of opportunity, 10, 11–13, 46, 128, 192, 211–12, 214–17, 224–5, 228–9; of results, 11–13; Sweden, 95

ethic, medical, 4, 48, 57, 70, 139–40, 151

expenditure, *see* costs, expansion

Family Practitioner Committee, Britain, 188

Fédération des Médecins de France (FMF), 139, 142, 146–7, 151–2, 153–4, 191

fee-for-service, 5–6, 89, 119, 125, 194; Britain, 188, 202; France, 144–7, 153, 156, 190–2; Germany, 187; US, 35–6, 40–2, 45, 51, 68–9, 71–2, 182, 204, 207, 225–6

Field, M., 181

Financial Survey of Health Care, Netherlands, 108, 109–10

financing of health care: Britain, 187, 201, 223–4; France, 152, 189; Germany, 159, 161–3, 165; Italy, 116, 121–2, 123–4, 127, 128–9; Netherlands, 100–2, 104, 110–11, 112–14; Sweden, 83, 87, 89, 193, *see also* budget financing

Flexner, Abraham, 34–5

France: medical autonomy, 15–17, 130–1, 139, 189–92, 196; political culture, 13, 14, 120, 133–7

Francesconi, D., 121

Freidson, Eliot, 6, 173, 198

Friedman, Milton, 21, 36

general practitioner (GP): as gatekeeper, 7, 187–9, 226; Netherlands, 100, 104; remuneration, 17, 20, 202

General Special Sickness Expenses Act 1967, Netherlands, 103, 105, 110–11

Germany, Federal Republic of: medical autonomy, 14–15, 126, 157, 173, 176, 184–7, 196; political culture, 13, 14, 120, 126–7, 157–61

GKV (social insurance), Germany, 159–61, 162, 174, 176, 184–5

GNP, health expenditure as share of, 1, 39, 76, 99, 132, 160, 200–1, 204, 223–5

goals, health care, 23–4, 32, 87, 93

Godt, P.J., 190, 191

Griffiths report, Britain, 206

Harrison, S., Pohlman, C. and Mercer, G., 5, 199

Haywood, S. and Alaszewski, A., 201–2

Health Care Cost Containment Act 1977 (KVKG), Germany, 162–4, 186

Health Care in the Eighties, Sweden, 87–8

Health Care Finance Administration (HCFA), 56, 59–69

Health Care Law 1962, Sweden, 93

Health Care in the Nineties, Sweden, 87–8

health maintenance programmes, US, 21, 43, 64, 183, 208–9

Health Planning Act 1974, US, 182

Health Services Act 1982, Netherlands, 104, 107–8, 113

Health and Sick Care Law 1982, Sweden, 86, 89, 90–4

Health Tariffs Act 1982, Netherlands, 108

Heidenheimer, A.J., 117, 193

Hill–Burton Act 1946, 39, 43, 45

Honigh, M., 112

hospital associations, Germany, 172–3

Hospital Cost Containment Act 1981, Germany, 162–4, 167

Hospital Facilities Act 1981, Netherlands, 103–7, 112–13

Hospital Financing Act 1972, Germany, 158–9, 161–3, 165–6, 168

Hospital Tariffs Act 1965, Netherlands, 102–4, 108

hospitals: France, 132, 141; Italy, 123, 127, 128; Netherlands, 100; Sweden, 76, 84, 89, 94–6, 192; US, 49–50, 56–7

Illich, Ivan, 179

in-patient care: Italy, 128; Netherlands, 104, 113; Sweden, 76, 77

incrementalism, 117, 118, 168

individualism, competitive, 10, 11–12, 21, 74, 118, 133

insurance: compulsory, 37–8, 120, 159–61, 184–5, 189, 192–3; national, 43–4, 47, 50–3, 71, 101, 103, 110, 113, 116, 121–2, 145, 182; private, 6, 35, 39, 51, 111, 120, 174, 182;

public, 6, 13, 16, 37–8, 39, 87, 161
interest groups, 109, 113–14, 158, 180; conflict
    paradigm, 210, 211–15, 218–20; France,
    134–5, 137–9, 142, 147–50, 152–4; *see also*
    associations, medical; centralization;
    consumer interests; professionals, medical;
    provider–consumer relations
intermediaries, fiscal, *see* US
intervention, public: comparative, 1–2, 5, 23,
    117–21; Europe, 12–13, 14–20, 21, 26,
    120–1; France, 16–17, 191–2, 196;
    Germany, 14, 162, 187; Netherlands, 15, 99,
    102–7, 111–14; organizational density, 6–7,
    26, 181–95; restriction, 50–1, 182–3;
    Sweden, 83–4, 86–8; US, 12–13, 21–2, 25–6,
    36–48, 52, 69, 120, 180, 205, 207, 216, 220
Italy: medical autonomy, 18–20; political
    culture, 11, 13, 14, 116–17, 121–5, *see also*
    national health service

Johnson, N., 198
judiciary, limited, France, 136–7, 149–50

Kelman, S., 17
KHG, *see* Hospital Financing Act
Klein, Rudolf, 179, 187, 189
Konzertierte Aktion, Germany, 164, 186,
    196–7
KV (*Kassenärztliche Vereinigung*), Germany,
    185–7
KVKG, *see* Health Care Cost Containment
    Act

Landau, M., 27
Länder, role of, 14, 158, 159, 161–4, 165–72,
    176–7
Landstingsförbundet (Federation of Swedish
    County Councils), 86–8, 90–1
leadership, doctors' role in, 5, 8–9, 48, 199
length of hospital stay: Britain, 206; France,
    132; Germany, 167, 169, 173–4; US, 42, 49,
    56–7, 59, 207
Levitt, R., 188
Lijphart, A., 99
litigation: Sweden; 85, US, 195, 202, 204–5,
    209
local government, 216; Sweden, 75–8, 78–83,
    85–7, 89–92, 94–7, 119–20, 193

McKeown, T., 179
McKnight, J., 70
management: Britain, 17, 202–3, 206; Italy,
    19–20, 129; Sweden, 18
market, *see* individualism, competitive
Marmor, T.R., 71, 182
médecine libérale, 144–5, 190–1
Medicaid, 21, 35–6, 46, 71, 120, 131, 182, 204;
    costs, 41–2, 44, 182
medical schools: Germany, 159, 175, 187; US,
    34–6, 48
Medicare, 21, 35–6, 46, 48, 57, 65, 68, 71, 120,
    131, 184, 204; AMA clause, 50–3, 182;
    costs, 38–9, 41–2, 44–5, 54, 58–62, 182, 207
Memorandum on the Structure of the Health
    Services, Netherlands, 103–4, 111, 113, 114
Mignot, G. and d'Orsay, P., 147
Millerson, G., 198
Mills, W., 51, 53, 58

monitoring of standards, 25, 42, 50, 54–8,
    183–7, 192, 208
monopoly of practice, 4, 21, 47–8, 50, 99, 139,
    200
Mosher, F., 28–9
Muntendam, P., 101

National Health Council, Netherlands, 15,
    104, 106, 107, 113–14
national health service: Britain, 17, 73, 119,
    187–8, 210; Italy, 18–20, 116, 121–9;
    Sweden, 18, 74–5, 117, 119–20, 192–5
negotiation, Sweden, 87–8, 93
Netherlands: medical autonomy, 15, 114;
    political culture, 13, 14, 99–100

occupancy rates, 132, 161, 163, 167, 172, 173
Oetzel, E.-A., 171
Olson, M., 138–9
organization, 23–4, 181–95; experimental,
    24–5; legal/bureaucratic, 23–4, 26
out-patient care: Germany, 174; Netherlands,
    113; Sweden, 75, 76, 89; US, 53, 68–9

participation, 19, 70, 125, 169, 219–20
particularism, 13, 16, 140, 141–2, 144, 147–8,
    153, 155
patient, rights, 48, 108, 199, 209
peer review, 22, 25–6, 195, 202–3; Sweden, 97;
    US, 22, 54–8, 75, 183, 203–4, 207–8
peer review organization (PRO), 42–3, 58–9,
    63–8, 72, 204, 208
performance: control, 1, 50; indicators, 206;
    system, 210–11, 213, 215, 224–7
Perkoff, G., 25
pharmaceutical industry, 123, 162
physicians, density: France, 141; Italy, 20,
    123; Sweden, 84, 119; US, 34–5, 72, 183,
    208–9, 227
Piperno, A., 121
planning: Bavaria and North Rhine
    Westphalia, 165–71; coordinating, 163–5;
    France, 147–55; Germany, 157, 159–60,
    162–75; Italy, 128; needs, 165–71, 174–6;
    Netherlands, 100–1, 103–4, 105–8, 112–14;
    professionals' input, 173–5; Sweden, 75, 76,
    85–8, 92, 97–8, 193; US, 41, 43, 72
pluralism: Germany, 160; US, 21, 26–7, 43,
    48, 61, 63, 66, 69, 72, 181–2
policy, comparative analysis, 10–22, 117–21
policy-making, *see* planning
prescribing, monitoring of, 189, 192, 206
preventive medicine, 8, 70, 87, 93, 103–4,
    127–8
price control, Netherlands, 101–2, 108–10
primary care, 76, 94, 103, 107, 192–3
private sector: Britain, 187–8, 200–2; France,
    156, 189; Germany, 172; Italy, 20, 125, 127,
    128; Netherlands, 99, 100–2, 107–8; Sweden,
    75–6, 94, 96, 192; US, 182
professional standards review organizations
    (PSROs), 22, 42, 54–8, 59–60, 62–8, 72,
    182, 204
professionals, paramedical, 8, 49, 195
professionals, medical, 3–4, 10, 22–7, 48,
    212–13; academic/non-academic, 78, 175;
    cohesion/fragmentation, 139–41; education
    and knowledge, 4, 28–9, 34–5, 36, 37,

48–50, 66, 139–40, 199; France, 120, 130–1,
137–56; Germany, 173–5; Italy, 121, 123,
126; Netherlands, 105, 108, 114; restriction
of entry, 4, 34–6, 131, 139, 187; status, 6,
17–18, 33, 130–1, 138, 179, 202; Sweden,
74–98; US, 182–4; *see also* associations,
medical; autonomy, medical; control,
political; general practitioners; specialists;
trade unions
provider–consumer relationship, 29–30, 31,
32–3, 37, 41, 48, 105, 133, 199, 212–15,
218–24
psychiatric care, Sweden, 76, 87
public, role in health politics, 31–3

quality of service: Britain, 203, 227–9;
Germany, 171; Netherlands, 107, 108, 111;
peer review, 25–6, 55–6, 58–9; and
remuneration, 5, 6; Sweden, 90, 95, 194;
US, 35–6, 39, 40, 51–2, 55–6, 63, 65–70,
182, 203–4, 227–9; and welfare state, 180–1
quangos: Britain, 188; Netherlands, 15, 104,
105–7, 110–11, 112–14

regionalization: Germany, 161–2, 164,
167–71; Italy, 19, 122–5, 126; Netherlands,
105; Sweden, 83, 94–8, 119
regulation, *see* intervention, public
remuneration: capitation, 6, 17, 20, 188–9,
196, 202, 208, 226; control over, 40–1, 45–6,
47–8, 58–9, 214–15; cost-based, 42, 47, 53,
58; France, 190–1; Germany, 171–3, 185–7;
prospective payment, US, 42, 45, 58–60,
62–3, 68, 184, 207; salary, 6, 17, 18, 89, 174,
188–9, 193–4, 196, 202, 225; Sweden, 75, 89,
193–4; *see also* fee-for-service
Republican Party (PRI), Italy, 122
resource allocation, 32, 72, 225; Germany,
158–9, 163–4, 166; public, 74–6; Sweden,
87–9, 94, 95–6; and welfare state, 178
Review Body for Doctors' and Dentists'
Remuneration, Britain, 188–9, 196
Rohde, J.J., 173

Saltman, R.B. and Young, D., 50
Salvati, M., 124
Schnabel, F., 173
sectarianism, 10–13, 17–20, 21
self-administration, sickness funds, 184–5
self-regulation, 30, 48, 52, 57, 65, 70, 133
Servizio Sanitario Nazionale, *see* national
health service, Italy
'seven crowns' reform, Sweden, 89, 119–20,
193–4
Sickness Fund Council, Netherlands, 15, 101,
104, 107, 110–11
sickness funds: France, 145–6, 152–3, 189–92;
Germany, 14, 160–3, 172–3, 176–7, 184–6;
Netherlands, 100–3, 110–11; Sweden, 192–4
Sickness Funds Insurance Act 1966, 103, 105,
110–11
Simon, H., 23
social security: France, 120, 132, 145, 152;
Italy, 121–2
Social Security Act (US), 40–3, 54, 62
Social Security Administration (US), 51–4
Socialist Party (PSI), Italy, 121–2
socialization of medicine, 119–20, 127–8,

187–8, 192–4, 196
specialists: Britain, 17, 188, 202; France,
140–1; Germany, 174–5; proliferation, 8,
28, 37, 100, 211–12, 222
specialization, Sweden, 95–6
SPRI (Institute for Health Planning and
Rationalization), 86, 88
standardization, 95, 127, 165, 213, 215–16
Starr, P., 37, 51, 184
Stevens, R., 227–8
strikes, administrative, 151
strikes, medical: France, 16, 147, 149–52, 155;
Italy, 20; Sweden, 18
Suleiman, Ezra N., 148–9, 153
supply, control, 104, 105–8, 131, 133
Sweden: medical autonomy, 81–3, 88, 89–90,
91–94, 97, 192–5; political culture, 13, 14,
74, 119–20, 127; *see also* national health
service
Swedish Medical Association, 89–91, 119,
193–4
syndicalism, France, 142–7

targeting, Italy, 128
tariffs, hospital, Netherlands, 100–3, 108–10,
112
Tax Equity and Fiscal Responsibility Act
1982, 42, 44–5, 58–9, 62
taxonomy, comparative, 3, 10–22, 181
technology, medical: and centralization, 7, 95,
222–3; cost, 1, 26, 132, 226–7; effectiveness,
1, 37, 131, 175, 227; and organizational
change, 212–13; and paramedical
professions, 8
Thiemeyer, T., 171
Tolliday, H., 199
trade unions: and health reforms, 121–2,
124–5; share in health service power, 2, 90,
114, 125

uncertainty, clinical, 65
unions, medical, *see* associations, medical
United Kingdom, *see* Britain
universalism, 13, 141
unpredictability, in service production, 49–50
US: fiscal intermediation, 6, 38, 39, 51–4, 71,
182; medical autonomy, 20–2, 28–37, 39–46,
47–56, 63, 71–2, 120, 131, 180, 182–3,
196–7, 207–9, 220; medical politics, 30,
33–46, 155, 181–4; political culture, 11–13,
26–7, 30–3, 120; *see also* intervention,
public
User Charges, Federal Regulations on
(BPflV), Germany, 161–2, 163, 171, 176–7
utilization rates, 166–7, 179, 206
utilization review, 22, 42, 50–4, 55, 56, 58, 59,
63–4, 66–9, 72, 207

waiting lists, 224–5, 228
welfare state, *see under* autonomy, medical
Wildavsky, A., 10–12
Wilson, F.L., 149–50

Zimmer, C.L., 172

*Index compiled by Meg Davies (Society of
Indexers)*

Notes on the Contributors

Christa Altenstetter is Professor of Political Science at the Graduate Center of the City University of New York as well as Queen's College. She has taught and researched at many other universities in the United States and in several European countries. Her books include *Federal–State Health Policies and Impacts* (co-author, 1978), *Innovation in Health Policy and Service Delivery: a Cross-National Perspective* (edited, 1981), and *Krankenhausbedarfsplanung* (1985).

Sven Arvidson teaches in the Department of Political Science at the University of Umeå, Sweden. Co-author of *Byråkrati och Förvaltning* (1986), his main interests lie in administration and the organization of health care systems.

Nico Baakman teaches public administration in the Department of Business and Public Administration of the Open University in Heerlen, the Netherlands. He has written on planning, normative aspects of the welfare state, and Dutch government policy on hospital construction.

James Warner Björkman is Director of the American Studies Research Centre, Hyderabad, India, as well as Executive Director of the International Institute of Comparative Government in Lausanne, Switzerland. He is also Clinical Professor of Preventive Medicine at the University of Wisconsin-Madison, USA, and has held other faculty appointments in Sweden, the UK, Pakistan, India and the USA. His books include *Federal–State Health Policies and Impacts* (co-author, 1978) and *The Politics of Administrative Alienation* (1979). He is currently (1985–90) conducting a major study of national health policies and politics in south Asia.

Marian Döhler is a Research Fellow at the International Institute of Management in Berlin, FRG. His research interests concern the German health care system and comparisons between health policies in the UK, the USA and the Federal Republic of Germany.

Maurizio Ferrera is Associate Professor of Italian Politics at the University of Pavia, Italy. While at the European University Institute in Florence he participated in an international research project, directed by Peter Flora, on the development of European welfare states since World War II. Among his publications are *Il Welfare State in Italia* (1984) and *La Salute che noi Pensiamo* (co-edited, 1986).

Giorgio Freddi is Professor of Public Policy and Chairman of the Department of Organization and Political Systems at the University of Bologna, Italy. He has held faculty appointments at several universities in the USA. He is Chairman of the Executive Committee of the European Consortium for Political Research and editor of *Rivista Trimestrale di*

Scienza dell'Amministrazione. His books include *Salute e Organizzazione nel Servizio Sanitario Nazionale* (1984) and *Manuale di Scienze dell' Amministrazione* (1988). His interests include health politics, comparative administration, methodology, organization theory, special purpose agencies, local government, and rational choice in administration.

Stephen Harrison worked as a personnel manager in the steel industry and the National Health Service before becoming Lecturer in policy services at the Nuffield Institute for Health Services Studies, University of Leeds, UK. His publications include *Health Services Performance* (co-edited, 1985), *Health Manpower Planning, Production and Management* (co-author, 1987), and *Managing the NHS in the 1980s* (1988).

J. Rogers Hollingsworth is Professor of History and Sociology at the University of Wisconsin-Madison, USA. His interests lie in the political economy of Western Europe and North America. Among his publications are *Centralization and Power in Social Service Delivery Systems* (1983) and *The Political Economy of Medicine: Great Britain and the United States* (1986).

Jan-Erik Lane is Professor of Public Administration at the University of Umeå, Sweden. Currently Chairman of the Committee on Conceptual and Terminological Analysis (COCTA), he has written extensively on comparative politics, political theory, public administration, and public policy. His recent publications include *Politics and Society in Western Europe* (1987) and *Bureaucracy and Public Choice* (edited, 1987).

Jan van der Made teaches politics and public administration in the Department of Health Sciences at the University of Limburg, the Netherlands. His recent publications focus on Dutch health care policy and on the political roles of interest groups.

Ingrid Mur-Veeman is Associate Professor on the faculty of Health Sciences at the University of Limburg, the Netherlands. She has also served as a policy adviser in health affairs for the provincial government of Brabant. Among other works on the Dutch health system and health legislation, she is author of *Ziekenhuisbeleid* (1981), on hospital policy-making.

Rockwell I. Schulz, a hospital administrator and management consultant before he entered university administration and teaching, is Founder-Director of the Health Services Administration Program, University of Wisconsin-Madison, USA, as well as the Wisconsin International Center for Health Services Studies. He is co-author of *Management of Hospitals* (1976, 1983) and *Teams and Top Managers in the National Health Service* (1983).

David Wilsford is Assistant Professor of Political Science at the University of Oklahoma, USA. His interests include the comparative politics of organized medicine in France, the UK and the USA. He is the author of *Organized Medicine, the State and the Corporation* (forthcoming).